PRAISE FOR *AM.*

"Alice Feller's *American Madness* is a personal memoir of her experience spanning almost 50 years of psychiatric practice. This important book documents the collapse of effective mental health care in America, which has led to inadequate treatment for a large part of the American population. The mental health system has become an ineffective treatment provider of the severely ill, the substance dependent, the poor, and racial minorities. This book is the work of a fine writer whose stories, while desperately sad, are written artfully in a way that reminds me of William Carlos Williams in his *Doctor Stories* and John Berger in *A Fortunate Man*. This is a must-read for all those who care about the repair of an insane system for treating the mentally ill." —**Thomas H. Ogden, MD, the Psychoanalytic Institute of Northern California; author of *Coming to Life in the Consulting Room* and *Reclaiming Unlived Life***

"This important and engaging book describes a complex national crisis through the lens of one thoughtful psychotherapist's life experience. Alice Feller has worked in almost every part of our fragmented mental health 'system.' Her book—part memoir, part policy discussion—helps the reader understand the causes of the crisis, the frustration of being a participant in a failing system, and what policy and program changes are needed to restore our communities to true mental health." —**Loni Hancock, former California State senator, California State assemblymember, mayor of Berkeley, and Berkeley City councilmember**

"Alice Feller's *American Madness* is a must-read if you're at all interested in the mental health crisis besetting this country. Dr. Feller embodies the staggering complexities of our system in vivid human stories. Her book is entertaining, illuminating, and absolutely necessary." —**David Schweidel, author of *What Men Call Treasure: The Search for Gold at Victorio Peak* and *Confidence of the Heart***

"I can't recommend *American Madness* enough. Alice Feller uses anecdotes drawn from her years of practice as a psychiatrist to convey, in a few strokes, the realities of serious mental illness, not only from the perspective of the provider but also in the experience of the patient. The writing is engaging and the vignettes flow smoothly in a way that is accessible and illuminating for the general public and those dealing with these issues in their own lives. She defines anosognosia, the inability by many with serious mental illnesses to have insight into their condition, in the clearest way I have seen. The personal narratives culminate in the final expository chapters, where Dr. Feller evaluates our mental health system and its failures. Most importantly, her heart and commitment to her patients comes through, and I wonder how different our outcomes might be if the system didn't make it so hard for these patient-first attributes to guide treatment." —**Patricia Fontana, activist and co-founder, Voices of Mothers**

"In *American Madness*, Dr. Alice Feller invites us on her decades-long journey through a shattered mental health system that is failing to treat our sickest, those with severe neurological brain diseases like schizophrenia and bipolar disorders. From when she began practicing medicine in 1977 to today, she recounts the step-by-step deterioration of a failing "system" in which people are blocked from urgently needed lifesaving medical treatment and are thereby denied the chance for a robust recovery.

"Dr. Feller's book addresses the many reasons we have let this population down, and she brings to light the frustrating obstacles dedicated, caring doctors now face to help their patients live their best lives. Her patients' poignant stories are recounted, bringing to life the avoidable human tragedies that continue to play out on our streets, in jail and prison cells, and in homes across our country.

"I highly recommend this thoughtful and compassionate recounting of a doctor's career in the trenches fighting for her patients' right to healthcare, dignity, and life." —**Linda L. Mimms, Public Policy, Duke University; vice chair, Schizophrenia & Psychosis Action Alliance**

AMERICAN MADNESS

AMERICAN MADNESS

Fighting for Patients in a Broken Mental Health System

ALICE FELLER, MD

ROWMAN & LITTLEFIELD

Lanham • Boulder • New York • London

Published by Rowman & Littlefield
An imprint of The Rowman & Littlefield Publishing Group, Inc.
4501 Forbes Boulevard, Suite 200, Lanham, Maryland 20706
www.rowman.com

86-90 Paul Street, London EC2A 4NE

British Library Cataloguing in Publication Information available

Library of Congress Cataloging-in-Publication Data
Names: Feller, Alice, author.
Title: American madness : fighting for patients in a broken mental health system / Alice Feller.
Description: Lanham : Rowman & Littlefield, 2024. | Includes bibliographical references and index.
Identifiers: LCCN 2023055862 (print) | LCCN 2023055863 (ebook) | ISBN 9781538193211 (cloth) | ISBN 9781538193228 (paperback) | ISBN 9781538193235 (epub)
Subjects: LCSH: Feller, Alice | Psychiatrists—United States—Biography. | Mental health services—United States—History. | Mental health policy—United States—History. | BISAC: PSYCHOLOGY / Mental Health | MEDICAL / Public Health
Classification: LCC RC438.6.F76 .F4 2024 (print) | LCC RC438.6.F76 (ebook) | DDC 616.890092 [B]—dc23/eng/20240301
LC record available at https://lccn.loc.gov/2023055862
LC ebook record available at https://lccn.loc.gov/2023055863

For Fred and Rebecca

In memory of Jessica, who fought her demons and won

CONTENTS

Expanded Contents

ACKNOWLEDGMENTS

A thousand thanks to Lilith Dorko at Rowman & Littlefield for her enthusiastic support of this project, to Jenna Dutton for her help with production, and to Kate Turner for introducing me to Rowman & Littlefield.

I am grateful to Scott Strain, Burt Dragin, and K. R. Nava at the *Laney Tower* for their advice and support during our weeklong media blast of homeless coverage and to Audrey Cooper, editor of the *San Francisco Chronicle*, for initiating that media event and opening our eyes to the history of homelessness.

I owe a huge debt of gratitude to my friends at FASMI for sharing their experiences and giving me a deeper understanding of life with a mentally ill family member, for their tireless advocacy on behalf of people suffering from severe mental illness, and for their companionship on our protest marches.

Thanks to David Schweidel for his reading and critique of an early version of *American Madness* and his helpful advice on writing and to all my friends in his class who read and commented on early pieces of this book.

I am immensely grateful to Scott Schaefer for his valuable insights, which changed this book for the better.

I could not have written the book without the help of my fellow writers Barbara Ridley, Claudia Marseille, Gail Kurtz, Lauren Cuttler, Jackson Lassiter, Irene Martinez, Holiday Jackson, Candis Cousins, and Josie Gallup, who read and critiqued so many parts of *American Madness* and gave me encouragement and invaluable advice.

Acknowledgments

Many thanks to Jess Walter at the 2013 Tin House summer workshop, who assured me that writing "takes the time it takes," and to Anthony Doerr, who lectured us with humor and compassion on the experience of failure.

Thanks also to Tony Johnson, Barry Braverman, Deborah and Bill Joost, Kate and Lowell Turner, Jim McEntee, Mary and Jake Smith, Hugh Robinson, and Paul Hapip for their fellowship and support of this project and to Mary Haake, who came to my rescue when it counted the most.

I will always be grateful to my sisters, Helen and Donna, for their reading and critiques of the manuscript and for their support.

A huge thank-you to my husband, Fred, for his many readings, helpful suggestions, and undaunted enthusiasm for this project.

Thanks also to my teachers at San Mateo Community Mental Health, UCSF, and SFPI, who helped me learn the art of psychotherapy.

And thank you to all my patients over the years who have taught me about the experience of mental illness.

INTRODUCTION

Long before I began my formal training as a psychiatrist, I wrote a high school term paper on schizophrenia in order to discover whether my father had this illness. I thought that if he did, he could get treatment and become normal, like other dads.

Years later, in 2017, I began writing the stories in this book. I'd taken a job as a staff psychiatrist in a mental health service center near San Francisco, where our patients suffered from severe mental illness. I wrote about the patients who stayed in my mind, the families I met, and the caseworkers who often became parent substitutes. I wrote about what moved me, but often I wrote about what shocked me.

Today the public is keenly aware that our mental health care system is broken, but despite large sums of money spent in good faith, it remains broken. We see the evidence of this on the streets, where people suffering from obvious mental illness make their home.

It wasn't always this way. In 1977, when I began my internship in psychiatry, I had the good fortune to work at Chope Hospital in San Mateo. It was part of a genuine community mental health program, the kind meant to replace our shuttered state mental hospitals. Our patients spent days, usually—or weeks at most—in that hospital, enough time to be stabilized and begin the process of recovery. It was a collaborative treatment model in which the nursing and medical staff met daily to coordinate the care of our patients. In addition, we psychiatrists coordinated patient care with our colleagues across the county. We had a fine nursing staff and a dedicated medical staff, large enough to pay close attention to each patient.

A few years later I worked at Highland Hospital in Oakland, where the shortage of beds was so severe that recovery was the rare exception. We had to discharge our patients almost as soon as they were admitted, long before they had a chance to become stable.

During the last 50 years, nearly all psychiatric hospitals—even the smallest local community hospitals—have closed. This came about largely due to an obscure law passed in 1965, the IMD exclusion, also known as the "16 bed rule." This law forbids the use of Medicaid (Medi-Cal in California) to pay for treatment in a psychiatric hospital with more than 16 beds. The purpose of the law was to close the large state hospitals and to save money. One result is that more than 90% of all inpatient psychiatric treatment today is provided in our prisons.

Although the IMD exclusion does not strictly apply to psychiatric wards located in general hospitals, these hospitals have been eliminating their psychiatric services, and there is no requirement that they continue to provide inpatient psychiatric care.

The IMD exclusion has also made residential substance abuse treatment unavailable to all but the very young, the very old, the very wealthy, or those with families willing and able to make huge sacrifices. Today's homeless and addiction crises have their roots in this law.

Meanwhile, racial discrimination continues with little change. Today African Americans suffer discrimination in health care, as well as more illness and early death. Through "weathering," a life of racial discrimination contributes directly to poor health. Surprisingly, the usual suspects—such as poor diet, lack of exercise, and smoking—contribute little. Mass incarceration as well as police violence are directed toward Black people far more often than white people and add their own brand of psychic trauma.

After many years away from public mental health care, mainly in private practice, my return was an eye-opening experience. I found that today, with the advent of electronic medical records (EMRs), the true mission of many facilities caring for people with severe mental illness is often just keeping the agency funded. We clinicians routinely spend as much time documenting service in our computers for the purpose of insurance billing as we do with our patients. This is insane.

Imagine if a carpenter had to stop his work every twenty minutes and fill out pages of computer forms so the contractor could be paid. Or if a chef had to stop her work and laboriously detail each meal so the restaurant could be paid. Yet in much of medicine, this approach is standard practice.

Fee for service, where each increment of treatment requires a separate insurance claim, sets up a cat and mouse game between the "providers" and the insurance entities, including Medicaid and Medicare. Transparency is rare, and each side suspects it's being cheated, which invites abuse on both sides. Insurance companies have found that they need not pay for mental health care.

"Up-coding" is the practice of writing in a more severe problem than the actual diagnosis, which bumps up the insurance reimbursement. I discovered that up-coding is widespread and standard practice in many areas of medicine, including the mental health clinics where I worked. Our patients suffer because the up-coded diagnosis often locks inappropriate treatment into place. For our clinic patients, it usually meant a diagnosis of schizophrenia, in many cases condemning them to years of treatment with powerful antipsychotic drugs and leaving them without the treatment that could actually help them.

In the first part of this book are vignettes showing our mental health system as it used to be, already fraying but nothing like the tattered scraps that remain today. Because homelessness, drug addiction, racial discrimination, and mental illness are often intertwined, I include chapters on the treatment of substance abuse, the history of homelessness, and the effects of racism.

The last half of this clinical memoir is taken from my recent work in our public mental health clinics. These are my patients' stories. I use their words to show the experience of severe mental illness, such as the voices that amplify their worst fears to bully and threaten them, often urging suicide. (The names and identifying features of all patients have been changed for reasons of confidentiality.)

I include vignettes that show the inner workings of today's fragmented mental health care system. One section features the board and care homes where many of our patients live today. I've included a number of stories showing the vital role of collaboration among coworkers, the numerous failures of such collaboration, and the sometimes deadly results that follow those failures. Several of these stories feature the mothers of my patients, who play a crucial role in helping their stricken children survive. At the end of the book, I've included suggestions for change.

This memoir is meant for anyone whose life is touched by mental illness, whether experienced personally or within the family. It's for policymakers, for all my colleagues in the mental health professions, and for anyone who wonders why our system is so broken and hopes to see it fixed.

Beginnings

A FAMILY AFFAIR

The first time my father threatened to start shooting, I was in the back-yard, playing in the sandbox with my two little sisters, digging out the moat for our castle. My mother burst out the back door, her face pale. In a shrill voice I'd never heard before, she said, "Come with me. *Now.*" She rushed us across the street to our friend Carmen's house, where we rang the doorbell then huddled on the doorstep, listening for footsteps inside. When Carmen opened the door and saw my mother's face, she whisked us inside. She settled the three of us children in the living room with a basket of blocks to play with and took my mother away to talk privately. While I strained to hear what my mother was telling Carmen, my sisters played happily with the blocks. But they were little. Helen was seven and Donna was only four. I was nine, and I worried.

After a long time, Carmen came out alone, her face grave. She placed her hands on my shoulders and looked me in the eye.

"Your father's just threatening," she said. "He's not really going to shoot himself."

Her words were hugely reassuring. I thought it was us he was going to kill. And as I imagined a life without him, I thought, *Go ahead. Shoot yourself. Let us be happy and safe.*

By that time, I was in third grade and could read the newspaper. I used to sit at the kitchen table after school, eating toast and reading the *Palo Alto Times*. It was full of news about Marilyn Monroe and

Khrushchev, who was threatening to drop his atom bomb on us. But the A-bomb didn't scare me. What did were the stories about men who shot their families and then themselves. I was afraid we'd be one of those families.

My sister Helen and I alerted each other to our father's moods with secret hand signals. A flat hand with fingers apart was "happy." Fingers together was "mad." We never put this into words—a questioning look was all it took. The answer was a quick flash of the hand, down low at the table so my father wouldn't see or out of sight in the kitchen.

His fury came out of the blue. Helen and I had the piano in our bedroom, and one day I was working on a Chopin prelude. I heard a door slam somewhere in the house, then the angry hiss of his slippers across the bare living room floor. I took my hands off the keyboard, trying not to look afraid. He burst into our room, slamming the door back against the wardrobe. As it wobbled forward on its hinges, he stood in the doorway, his face white with fury.

"I don't *ever* want to hear that *insipid drivel* again—you got that?"

I looked at him silently till he turned away. When he slammed the door behind him, the walls vibrated.

I never played Chopin again when he was home. Or anything else. Not the Bach he loved or Mozart. Playing the piano was my portal into a private world where I could feel and be all those things I wasn't in my real life. Tiptoeing around to avoid displeasing him would turn it into a joyless exercise. I'd practice in the afternoon, and as soon as I heard his car in the garage, I would stop.

As with other families who cope with the insanity of one member, his emotional disturbance had a profound effect on each of us. We adjusted our behavior to accommodate his paranoia and to be ever ready for his unpredictable rages. We tried to pretend we weren't scared, when really, we were. We tried to keep his insanity a secret, which left us isolated from the outside world. My mother had few friends and turned to me for advice when things got scary.

Without ever speaking about it, my sisters and I made sure to get our friends out of the house before he came home from work. Normal people, who were unaware of all we did to avoid making him mad, would treat him in the casual and friendly way acceptable in other households. But he took offense easily. If we hadn't managed to get our friend out of the house in time, he might find some reason to explode into a frightening rage. Then our friend would witness our family insanity.

We lived in the quiet and orderly town of Palo Alto. Our street was lined with perfect lawns in front of every house, except for ours. At my father's insistence, we guarded our front lawn behind a cyclone fence on two sides and a wide swath of prickly juniper separating it from the sidewalk. At some point I knew it was weird. We were the odd shipwreck in a fleet of normalcy.

Then one day, as I was walking home from school, I witnessed a scene I never forgot. There was a red house near the end of our block, fronted by a perfect lawn like all the rest. I knew the children by sight—pale, silent kids I'd seen on the playground at school. But I'd never seen the parents or any of the family out in front of the house. That was unusual for this neighborhood.

But that day, as I walked by, the front door burst open and a small boy raced out of the house onto the perfect lawn, pursued by his raging mother, who grabbed him and dragged him back inside. It was 3 o'clock in the afternoon and she was wearing a bathrobe. Something about her fury, the bathrobe, and the beaten-down air of those kids formed a picture in my mind. Here was another family that hid its craziness behind closed doors, I thought. We weren't the only ones.

WESTERN PSYCH

A year after *One Flew over the Cuckoo's Nest* swept the Oscars, I found myself in a large psychiatric hospital, on a locked ward with bars on the windows. I came as a medical student.

I was intensely curious about this hospital, having seen *Cuckoo's Nest* and all the horrors it portrayed. I'd seen how Nurse Ratched tortures the shy young man who seems to have nothing wrong with him beyond a kind of adolescent insecurity. I was prepared to see patients being abused in group therapy.

Most of all, I was anticipating with dread the "shock therapy" I'd seen in that movie. After all his bravado, Jack Nicholson is unable to hide his terror in that memorable scene and is held down by six large men while he is shocked, wide awake and enduring this vicious torture by order of Nurse Ratched, to punish him for insubordination. *Cuckoo's Nest* told us these are the crimes against humanity carried out behind the locked doors of psychiatric hospitals.

The ward was on the ninth floor of Western Psych in Pittsburgh, Pennsylvania. It was the summer of 1976, and I was doing my six weeks of psychiatry before resigning myself to internal medicine. It was the moment that each of us medical students chose which direction to go after graduation—most were deciding among surgery, internal medicine, pediatrics, or obstetrics and gynecology.

It felt as if we were choosing who we'd be for the rest of our lives. I knew I'd like psychiatry, but it was out of the question. *Cuckoo's Nest* and other movies like it had painted a vivid picture of psychiatrists as idiot weaklings and cruel into the bargain. I didn't want to be seen that way. And I'd watched for eight years as the useless Dr. Ross saw my parents in couples therapy, which was supposed to help my father. It helped my mother, but my brilliant father couldn't hold a job. As he got crazier, no one wanted to work with him. Angrily I agreed. Psychiatrists were a bunch of feckless fools. That would never be me.

We could go for prestige—surgery was the "coolest" choice. Or we could go for intellect—that would mean internal medicine. But it was the end of our third year, the deadline to make up our minds. We acted as if we were full of certainty, and then let loose with a barrage of jokes, such as: *The surgeon knows nothing and does everything. The internist knows everything and does nothing. The pathologist knows everything and does everything, but it's too late.*

I assured my classmates I was going for internal medicine.

But the medical wards were heavy with despair and the anguish of prolonged dying. I remember hearing screams from a patient's room, a woman whose tumor was eating into her bones. I heard an old man begging a team of young doctors to leave him alone as they readied their instruments and closed the green curtain around his bed.

And a peculiar odor hung over those floors. It hit you when you stepped out of the elevator. Later I realized it was the smell of slow death.

At Western Psych I'd step off the elevator onto the ninth floor, look up through the wire mesh window as I turned the key to let myself onto the ward, and see my patient, Rochelle, rushing the door. Not to escape but to talk.

Rochelle was 20 years old, stuck in the hospital, and longing to get back to her real life. Every day she made her case to me that she was ready to leave. I agreed because I liked her and saw how desperate she was to go home. And I didn't see why she was in the hospital. So every day I listened while she told me about her love life. It was my favorite hour of the day. Afterward, I would argue her case for discharge to the attending doctor, who shook her head as soon as I began. "She's not ready. She'll embarrass herself."

I always bristled at that. Rochelle was thoroughly charming, bursting with life. She had energy to spare and was always in high spirits. Her words burst out as if shot from a fire hose, and she jumped from one story to another so that often that I was confused. But her mood was contagious, and I loved listening to her. I didn't like to think that she was in an altered state, one that could distort her sense of reality and impair her judgment.

In the "history of present illness" in her medical record for this hospitalization, I'd read that she had a history of "manic depressive illness" (bipolar disorder) and that she was currently in the midst of a manic episode. Like others in this state, she needed very little sleep and was charged with a booming self-confidence not always based in reality.

People amid a manic episode are apt to make impulsive decisions that later turn out to be disastrous. Sudden marriages and unwise business decisions are common, along with multiple bankruptcies and divorces. To understand how one person can accomplish such a life, it's important to understand that bipolar disorder is cyclic. In between acute episodes of depression or mania, people are well and live normal, often very successful lives. We don't use the term much these days, but we used to talk about "hypomania." This term describes the high-energy, confident, and outgoing personality in people between acute episodes of this illness. As with my patient Rochelle, this delightful mood is contagious. It helps people make new friends, start new businesses, and fall in love again, which helps me understand the frequent history of multiple bank-ruptcies and divorces.

Rochelle hadn't reached this happy state yet. Even as she charmed me with her high spirits and her stories, her speech was pressured and often tangential, sometimes jumping from one story to another completely unrelated story, leaving me struggling to follow her train of thought.

Occasionally people in the throes of a manic episode become psy-chotic, with delusions and even hallucinations. In the emergency room, it's hard to tell whether this is an acute psychotic episode of schizophre-nia, an acute manic episode due to bipolar disorder, a drug-induced state due to a stimulant drug such as methamphetamine, or an acute psychotic state caused by an underlying medical illness.

In the ER—or with any unfamiliar patient in a state of psycho-sis—medical records are invaluable. A useful medical record, one meant for patient care rather than insurance billing, contains a record of past treatment. For every hospitalization, there is a social history including marriages, children, occupation, and work history. Multiple episodes of illness with long periods of high functioning in between episodes suggest bipolar disorder rather than schizophrenia. The other telling piece of his-tory is the patient's age at first episode. People with schizophrenia usually become sick in their teens or early twenties. But a first manic episode can occur at any age. In either case, the onset of illness is often precipitated by a stressful event.

I had a patient in her fifties who was hospitalized after a personality change and the onset of wild behavior that was completely out of char-acter for her. After having a few drinks at a local bar, she climbed onto the counter and danced for the whole room. She told me she'd entered into a strange and completely uncharacteristic mood after a shocking experience. She had gone upstairs and discovered her beloved husband, sitting up in bed but no longer alive.

The other pole of bipolar disorder is depression. Those affected often suffer episodes of severe depression as well as manic states. The depres-sion in this illness is often so deep and convincing that suicidal thoughts and wishes, sometimes acted on, are common. In my experience, this mood, too, is contagious. The afflicted person moves slowly and speaks haltingly if at all. For me, it feels as if the room has gotten dark, the air heavy with despair. The patient feels hopeless, self-blaming, and fearful.

Today we have mood stabilizers for bipolar disorder, medications that can prevent the manic episodes altogether and help to prevent the depressive episodes as well.

The first mood stabilizer to be developed was lithium carbonate, a breakthrough in the treatment of this often-disabling illness. Lithium is burdensome to use, as it requires repeated blood work to ensure the correct dosage: by measuring the lithium concentration in the blood. There is a rather narrow therapeutic range, below which the drug is ineffective, and above which kidney damage can occur. To guard against this danger, we also get blood work to monitor kidney function. A common side effect of lithium is a mild tremor. Today we have other mood stabilizers, including anticonvulsants (used originally to prevent seizures) such as Depakote.

For severe depression, we had antidepressants, which in those days were so loaded with side effects that it often took months to get onto a therapeutic dose of the right drug. For faster results, we had ECT (electroconvulsive therapy), known to the rest of the world as "shock therapy."

I remember escorting my first patient, Mr. Hawthorn, to the little ECT station. Remembering the shock therapy scene in *Cuckoo's Nest*, I dreaded what I would see. My poor patient would writhe in pain, arms and legs jerking spasmodically while six strong men held him down. His hair would stand on end and after it was over his scalp would be covered with burns from the electrodes. I worried that I might be recruited to help hold him down and recoiled at the thought.

When we got to the station, there was only the doctor, who had my patient lie on the table, and a nurse anesthetist, who started an IV. She had him count backward till he fell asleep and then intubated him and breathed for him with an inflatable rubber bag, and I realized he was getting general anesthesia for the procedure, as if he were having surgery.

The doctor fastened electrodes on either side of his forehead to induce a grand mal seizure and turned the dial on his instrument, a small box about the size of a radio. My patient lay completely still, except for a twitch in one of his big toes. Then it was over.

I knew the seizure is what relieves depression, not the electricity itself. In the past, insulin was used to induce a grand mal seizure. But patients suffered unbearable feelings of dread as their blood sugar plummeted. ECT was found to be safer and more humane. Nobody explained how a grand mal seizure works to free the patient from a severe depression; it just did. I always imagined it as something like pressing "reset" on a video game or shutting down a computer to get rid of the accumulated bugs.

When Mr. Hawthorn woke up from the anesthetic, he'd lost his memory of everything from the past day due to the seizure in his brain. He was so confused he couldn't remember how to get back to his bed. My job was simply to lead him back that short distance. Over the next couple of days, he began to remember things again. Meanwhile, I thought how different the scene in *Cuckoo's Nest* was from the real thing.

We saw a film about another man who had ECT at Western Psych. It was screened for us by my favorite teacher, Alan Meisel, who taught courses on psychiatry and the law. He was investigating whether it was possible to give informed consent amid a psychotic episode (Lidz et al., 1984).

One day he showed us a film of an interview he'd done with a severely depressed patient who agreed to be in his study. The old man hunched under a rough blanket, staring at Meisel with a blank, terrified look. His wife sat close to him with her eyes fixed on his face, as if she could will him to be better.

Meisel spoke to him in easy sentences, his pace gentle. He recommended ECT for his depression and explained what it was and why he thought it would help. When he asked the patient if he wanted to have this treatment, the old man whispered, "Yes." He nodded jerkily as if to urge the interview to an end.

"Do you have any questions?" Meisel asked.

The old man looked blank and his wife whispered to him. He nodded his head in the same hurried manner. *Just get me out of here*, he seemed to say.

After that, Meisel turned on the lights and told us the rest of the story. The patient did have a course of ECT and it relieved his depression. When they met again and Meisel asked if he remembered that first interview, the old man said of course he did. But he thought he was refusing the treatment. In fact, his severe depression had so confused him that he was unable to follow the conversation, including his own part in it.

The outcome could be seen as fortunate, because the treatment relieved his disabling illness and brought him back to his usual self. But was he able to properly give consent? Informed consent by a person in a state of psychosis is a hotly debated topic today, because it includes informed refusal of treatment as well as agreement to treatment.

Meisel went back to the law school to teach his fall courses. Rochelle got through her manic episode and went home. The ward was flatter and sadder without her. It was time for me to bite the bullet and apply for internal medicine internships.

On one of my last days at Western Psych, I rode the elevator to the ninth floor as usual. A blast of Motown music hit me as I let myself onto the unit. Bobbie had his portable record player out in the middle of the floor and next to it a stack of 45s. He was 18 years old, flamboyantly gay, and dressed in his own high fashion. Eyes closed, he swayed and gyrated to the music.

Watching Bobbie, it hit me that I could choose a different path, too. I chose with my heart and went into psychiatry.

Community Mental Health

PSYCH EMERGENCY

I went off the beaten path for my internship and residency, choosing a small program in San Mateo County, just south of San Francisco. What attracted me to this program was its experimental group home, where people suffering from severe psychosis lived together without benefit of medication. I wanted to be like Dr. Fried, in *I Never Promised You a Rose Garden*, who cured the author of that book through talk therapy alone (Greenberg, 1964).

Unfortunately, the experiment was not a success and was halted after one of the house's residents drowned another resident in the bathtub. By the time I arrived, everyone in that house was on medication.

I was lucky to land there anyway. San Mateo County had a genuine community mental health care system, the kind that had been promised when the large state hospitals were closed. At the time I didn't appreciate how excellent and unusual our program was. I thought that every psychiatric hospital would have beds for the people who needed them, would provide them with good care, and would arrange for housing after discharge if necessary. I thought that our collaboration with others in the county system was standard and that my patients would always have good outpatient care in one of our clinics after leaving the hospital.

In the beginning, though, the place scared me. It brought to mind "The Adventure of the Speckled Band," a Sherlock Holmes story I'd heard as a child, in which the murderer arranges for the death of his houseguest by positioning his bed beneath a seemingly innocent grate in the ceiling. At night a venomous snake—the speckled band—drops through the grate and bites the victim (Conan Doyle, 1892). The thing about that bed was that it was bolted to the floor.

When I began my internship, I saw another bed bolted to the floor. It was in the back of the locked room at the Chope Hospital ER in San Mateo, where I was a brand new intern. The people who ended up in that locked room were brought by the police on a 5150 psychiatric hold. On nights when I was the intern covering the ER, it was my job to examine the patient and determine whether the hold was warranted. The "5150" is a 72-hour involuntary hold based on evidence that the person is "a danger to self, a danger to others, or gravely disabled" due to a mental illness not caused by drugs or alcohol. "Gravely disabled" is defined as being unable to provide for one's own food, clothing, and shelter or to accept it from others.

I would read the cop's brief statement on the 5150 form, read through past medical records brought up from the chart room, and interview the patient. If I agreed that the hold was warranted, I would write my own 5150 document, detailing all the evidence supporting that decision.

If, on the other hand, I didn't think the patient was "holdable," I would document every shred of evidence that supported my decision not to renew the hold. Many times I wondered, in some small corner of my mind, whether it was really safe to let a patient go, whether I was missing something. If my decision resulted in injury or death, it would be a calamity, something I'd have to live with for the rest of my life. But I couldn't justify keeping someone who didn't seem to pose a real danger to himself or others.

Most of our patients were voluntary, not on a hold, and I would find them in the waiting room. Otherwise I had to start our conversation in the locked room.

That room was always dim, with no light except what came through the little observation window in the locked door. It was bare except for the iron bed bolted to the concrete floor.

Usually the patients were free to roam around that room, but sometimes paramedics would arrive with the cops and wheel the patient into the ER on a gurney in restraints. Then they would transfer him to the bed in the locked room, which also had restraints—large leather straps that buckled around their wrists and ankles. A nurse, acting on standing orders and always unseen by us residents, would inject the patient with 5 milligrams of Haldol. This powerful antipsychotic drug helps to quiet the terror and hallucinations our psychotic patients suffer so that they can think more clearly.

I thought it was an advantage that I was a woman. It was always a man who ended up in restraints, so the patient on the bed was still the only man in the room. I thought it helped, too, that I was a small woman. I'd go in quietly, introduce myself, and approach as gently as I could.

Five milligrams of Haldol would put most people to sleep, but I don't remember anyone falling asleep. As I walked the length of that long room, I always had the full attention of the man on the bed.

"How're you doing?" I'd say. I'd ask him what happened.

If we could have any sort of conversation, I'd ask if we could move to my office across the hall. No one ever refused. My colleagues differed on whether to keep the office door open (for safety) or closed (for privacy). I always closed the door. How can you expect people to tell you anything if you leave the door open, with other people walking up and down the hall outside the office? Nothing bad ever happened. Even when I ended up telling a patient I was going to keep him in the hospital, no one ever did anything to hurt me. I was never afraid that they would.

The patients were the ones who were frightened, I think. After we finished talking, I'd do a brief physical exam. When I listened to the patient's heart with the stethoscope in my right hand, I'd rest my left hand on the patient's shoulder and hear their heart rate slow down. That was my favorite moment.

What I hated was the locked room. I hated being a jailer. One night, Mr. Walker, a new patient, provided a fresh experience of what that meant.

It was close to midnight when he arrived, strapped to a gurney in four-point restraints. As the paramedics wheeled him past my open door opposite the locked room, he watched me with casual calm. He looked like Rasputin, long boned and black haired, with a pale face and eyes that bore into mine.

"He has a head injury," the cop told me as he slapped the paperwork down on the counter of the nurses station. "Just so you know."

The paramedics returned from the locked room, the empty gurney rattling along as they passed. "Head injury," one of them called. "Make sure you read the face sheet."

At the nurses station, I stood and read the 5150 form. Mr. Walker was being held as a "danger to others" and "danger to self." On the form, the cop had written, "Subject armed with a lead pipe, claimed he was hunting vampires." They didn't spell it out, but I imagined a struggle. Most likely one of them had clubbed him over the head with his baton or his heavy flashlight in the effort to subdue him. Ordinarily Mr. Walker would have gotten a dose of Haldol as soon as he arrived. But with the head injury, we needed him to stay alert in case he was bleeding inside his skull.

In med school, we were warned about this sort of injury with an anecdote about a high school baseball player who was hit in the head with a wild pitch. He walked off the field with a headache, refused all medical treatment, and went home to bed. In the morning, his mother found him dead.

It turned out he had a skull fracture. During the course of the night, he bled into the closed space between his skull and his brain, the blood pooling until it forced his brain stem down through the large opening at the base of his skull. The nerves running through his brain stem were crushed, one by one. When the nerves serving his diaphragm gave out, he stopped breathing.

My job would be to watch Mr. Walker and determine whether he seemed to be bleeding into his skull. The first signs would be headache and decreased level of consciousness. Then there would be changes in his eyes: a dilated pupil on one side that didn't react to light, then trouble following the light with his eyes. But I wasn't going to let it get anywhere close to that point. If he got groggy, I'd call for a medical consult.

I took my penlight and let myself into the locked room. It was dim, lit only from the light outside in the hall. Mr. Walker watched me through the gloom as I approached and introduced myself.

"How are you feeling?" He held my gaze but said nothing. "I understand you got hit on the head. Are you in pain?" More silence. "I'm going to take a look. Is that all right?" He watched me in silence while I felt for lumps or blood. He had a swelling over one ear but nothing more.

His pupils constricted equally and briskly in the light and he moved his eyes smoothly to follow my finger.

"Great. Can you tell me about what happened this evening?"

He fixed his eyes on me but said nothing.

"Okay, maybe later. I'll check back with you in a while."

I had no idea when I should check again. It all depended on how fast the blood might be pooling. If it was pooling.

So if the ballplayer's mother had checked him at dinnertime, would he have been groggy but still alive? Maybe he was already dead by dinnertime. What if she had checked him after an hour?

I got out my *Washington Manual* (Boedecker and Dauber, 1973), the battered book we all lugged around in the giant pockets of our white coats. Supposedly it contained everything the intern needed to know to get through a night on call. It described the mechanics of this injury but gave no clues about how often to check the patient. I called radiology to see if someone could come to the locked room with a portable X-ray machine. Not possible, said the X-ray tech. In the end, I decided one hour would be soon enough.

It felt horrible to leave him in restraints. I wanted to take them off, but what if I did and he became violent again? If only he would talk to me, I could gauge the risk.

After an hour he was the same. Wide awake, eyes perfect, unspeaking.

"Can you tell me what happened?"

Again, he only stared at me. He seemed so alert I decided to wait two hours before checking him again and went upstairs to the on-call room for a fruitless attempt at sleep. At 3:00 a.m., I went back down to see him again.

For me, 3:00 a.m. was the witching hour. The lights were low, and the ER was deserted. It felt creepy in a way it hadn't before. Again Mr. Walker was completely alert, with a normal exam. But this time when I tried to speak with him, he seemed to be responding. He moved his lips and made a barely audible sound.

At last. Finally we were going to talk. I wanted to know this strange man and hear his story. Was he really out hunting vampires? A feeling of gratitude, almost love, washed over me.

"Could you speak a little louder?"

He motioned with his head for me to come closer and I bent down to hear him. Then with a sudden movement, his jaws open wide, he lunged at my neck. I jumped back, my heart pounding. As if he could burst out of the restraints, rise up off the bed, and grab me, I fled out the door, heaved it closed behind me, and turned the lock. When I looked back through the wire mesh window, I saw he was laughing.

It wasn't very professional of me, but all my sympathy for him evaporated.

I didn't think he was bleeding inside his skull. He was completely alert, alert enough to play that trick on me. The next time I waited longer, almost till morning, before going down again. He began speaking right away.

"I thought you were the nurse," he said.

As if that would make it okay, I thought. "Just watch the light."

His pupils were equal and reactive. "When the day shift comes on, security will take you up to X-ray and get skull films."

Then I left the room, feeling derelict in my duty. I should have stayed and gotten some history now that he was talking. But I'd had enough of the vampire man.

Fortunately, after Mr. Walker was admitted to the psychiatric ward upstairs, he became another intern's patient, not mine. I never did learn his diagnosis. Why he ended up threatening people with a lead pipe was a mystery. Perhaps he was psychotic and really thought there were vampires to slay, but he seemed to be clear-headed, not hallucinating or delusional.

Three weeks later, a new patient came into the ER, a young woman on a 5150 as a danger to herself. According to the brief history on the intake sheet, the highway patrol had found her wandering beside the freeway, trying to cross traffic to get onto the median strip. She told them there were "people after her." Also, she said she was a marathon runner. Now she was in the locked room.

Before we went into that room, we followed a set routine: look through the wire mesh window into the room, call to the patient to let them know you're coming in, and make sure they're sitting on the bed before you go in. I walked across the hall to look through the little window at my new patient. She was young and fragile looking. She paced in tight circles around the narrow room. She looked so harmless and vulnerable that I forgot all about having her sit on the bed.

"Hi," I called. "I'm the doctor. I'm coming in to talk with you."

As I opened the door and stepped into the room, she stopped and stared at me for an instant. Then she turned to some invisible person beside her and cried, "Run for your life!" She sped past me out the door I'd left ajar, rounded the front desk, and was out the double glass doors, racing through the parking lot.

Three blocks away was El Camino Real, four lanes of fast-moving traffic. I could imagine her dashing out in front of a speeding car as she fled from whatever was pursuing her. I raced after her, calling to the startled unit clerk for backup as I hurtled through the glass doors and out to the parking lot. We must have made quite a sight running through that sedate San Mateo neighborhood: two women in street clothes, one fleeing and the other pursuing.

After seven or eight blocks, we came to a large RV parked along the sidewalk, and my patient disappeared around the front of it. Cautiously I circled the opposite way until we faced each other from a safe distance. Both of us were breathing hard. I leaned against the RV and felt the sweat running down my face.

"Tell me about these people who are after you," I gasped.

She watched me warily, still catching her breath. But she didn't run away.

Finally the hospital security guard drove up in his gray county car to collect us. We rode sitting side by side in the back seat, like two prisoners in a squad car. But I didn't care. I hadn't lost my patient and nothing else mattered.

Ward 2N

Ward 2N, upstairs from the ER, was where three of us interns began our residencies. It was Walter, the chief of psychiatry, who showed me around the ward that first day. All of us, patients and staff, ate together at a long table that ran down the center of the ward. He showed me our breakfast: scrambled eggs and soggy hash browns, sent up by the hospital kitchen in big metal pans, kept warm on a hot plate in the back of the ward. After we'd filled our plates and found seats at the long table, Walter started a comfortable banter with a patient across from us. Something in the cadence of his rumbling voice seemed to reassure the man. He raised his head with new life in his face and I relaxed.

An air of kindness mingled with the chaos and suffering that brought our patients there. Our charge nurse, Hazel, was a motherly presence for us greenhorn interns. In her large desk with its many drawers, she'd always find whatever I asked her for. And she never made me feel dumb about asking for it.

The marathon runner became my patient on Ward 2N. She went by Betsy, she told me. I noticed she was 33 years old, older than I was. She seemed so young and helpless; it startled me and made her more mysterious. Ordinarily, her old chart would have come up from Medical Records, and before seeing her, I would have sat in the nurses station reading discharge summaries from earlier hospitalizations or notes from prior ER visits. But she'd never been seen at Chope Hospital before, so she had no old records.

All we had was the blue three-ring binder with our notes from her current hospitalization. It held the nursing intake notes, my own notes from the ER, and the cop's history on the 5150 form. The highway patrol had spotted her by the side of the freeway. Something was coming after her, she told them.

When I sat down with her that first morning on the ward, she told me she'd been working as a hair stylist for five years. She couldn't explain how she happened to be walking next to the freeway, except to say she was trying to get onto the freeway median, where she'd be safe.

"Do you feel safe here?" I asked.

We were sitting out on the deck. It was a warm October day, the Bay breeze just enough to keep us cool. She turned to look at the screen that enclosed the deck, seeming to listen for something.

I waited, watching her and noticing again how very thin she was. In the bright sunlight, I could see the outline of bones under her pale skin.

Finally she turned back and gave me a quick glance. "I guess so." Her voice was tiny and far away.

"You don't sound so sure," I said. "What's worrying you?"

She took a moment to answer, then leaned toward me, speaking in a low voice. "Werewolves. I hear them howling."

"Yikes. That sounds terrifying."

"I see their yellow eyes in the window at night. They watch me when I get undressed."

Under "Assessment" in my chart note, I wrote, "rule out schizophrenia, rule out bipolar disorder, manic episode." But she was so frightened, I knew she wasn't manic. She'd worked as a hair stylist for five years, and at 33, she was a little old for a first episode of schizophrenia.

I brought her up during rounds the next morning. We met in Walter's office, and it was a tight squeeze, with Walter, Hazel, our psych tech, and the three of us interns jammed together on folding chairs. Nobody else thought Betsy was schizophrenic, either. Not Hazel, with her long experience of treating psychotic patients, and not Marty, our veteran psych tech.

"She sees their yellow eyes, watching her from the window," I told them.

"Amphetamine psychosis," Walter said, and the others nodded. "Visual hallucinations and paranoid delusions." He agreed to let me hold off on antipsychotic drugs. If she got better with no medication, that would point to drug toxicity, not schizophrenia.

19

Hospitalization is generally helpful for people with acute episodes of psychosis. In the safety of the hospital, we can let any street drugs clear from their systems. Sometimes this is all that's needed.

If they were stable on an antipsychotic medication but stopped taking it, we have to ask why they stopped it. Sometimes people suffer side effects that feel worse than the illness itself. It's important for us to know this so that we can find a medication that works better for them. Often people stop their medication for reasons unrelated to the drug itself but due to what it means to take such a drug or because it's difficult to stay on a routine.

If they're willing, we can start them back on the same medication and hope it relieves their symptoms. If it doesn't, we have to try a different drug, the same drug at a different dose, or perhaps even a different class of drugs. People with bipolar disorder, for instance, need mood stabilizers rather than antipsychotics.

In the hospital, we meet with our patients every day, and we can ask about side effects as well as therapeutic effects. Are the hallucinations quieting? Does the world feel less threatening? Is the drug causing unpleasant side effects? And always, we have the benefit of a whole team—other doctors, nurses, and psych techs—who work in shifts around the clock to help us with their observations.

Betsy denied any drug use, and after three days, her 5150 was about to run out, but she was still frightened, confused, and hallucinating. We were outside on the terrace, where it was quiet and we could talk in private.

"You came here on a hold," I reminded her. "But this is day three and that hold runs out today. How would you feel about staying for a couple more days? Till you feel like your old self?"

She looked startled. "I've been here three days?"

"Yes. So what do you think—would you be okay with staying for a couple more days?" I watched her face, hoping she'd agree.

"I guess."

"Great. We'll need you to sign in as a voluntary patient."

"Okay."

I was relieved. If she had refused, I was going to petition for a 14-day certification so we could treat her a little longer, but I didn't want to keep her as an involuntary patient if I didn't have to.

Two days later, the werewolves were gone and she seemed more relaxed. Then she told me about the Ritalin. Later medications such as Adderall have since replaced it, but at that time Ritalin was widely used to treat hyperactivity in children. "It's supposed to help me concentrate. But I save it up and have a party. No sleep for days." She laughed and then caught my eye. "I guess I should throw it out."

"That would be a good idea," I said. "Do you feel ready to go home?"

Betsy went home that afternoon and I never saw her again. But other patients we saw over and over again. When they came onto the ward, they were greeted with affection by the staff. Their old charts, when they came up from Medical Records, were thick and heavy.

I was the intern covering psych emergency one day when one of those fat charts landed on my desk. I flipped it open to look at the face sheet and saw that the patient's name was Jeff Bryant. I did a double take, hoping it wasn't the same boy I knew from grade school.

That Jeff Bryant was a year ahead of me, but we all knew who he was. People called him JB. He'd walk the red tile corridors outside our classrooms, always surrounded by friends, unmistakable even from behind with his pale blond hair. At recess he was picked first for kickball, and when he was up, I'd stop to watch. He would kick the ball far out over the field and lope gracefully around the bases to tag home plate. If he happened to catch my eye he'd give me his aw-shucks grin.

Trying to look casual, I walked out to the waiting room to see if he was the same boy. He was. A man now, but unmistakably the same JB. In shock, I retreated to my office and closed the door. I needed a minute of privacy to collect myself. Then I looked at his chart, hoping against hope that his diagnosis wouldn't be schizophrenia. But it was.

By then I'd been thinking about schizophrenia for half my life, ever since tenth grade, when I'd written a term paper on the topic. I was hoping to find out if my father had this illness. If he did, I thought, he could be treated. Then we wouldn't have to be afraid of him.

I learned that schizophrenia is common. One out of every hundred human beings on earth is afflicted with this illness. It affects rich and poor equally. Good parenting doesn't prevent it, and bad parenting doesn't cause it. It strikes early in life, often in adolescence.

To my great disappointment, I saw right away that my father didn't have schizophrenia. He never had hallucinations, never heard voices. Although he was suspicious and paranoid, he wasn't actually delusional. Many people shared his belief that the Communists in far-off Vietnam were a threat to us Americans. I thought that was crazy, but I knew it didn't qualify as delusional. Although he was losing jobs, he hadn't fallen apart and become unable to function. He didn't act bizarre, just embarrassing. He yelled at my mother and us kids, but he didn't yell at imaginary people that no one else could see.

When I went out to the waiting room to meet JB, I wondered if he would recognize me, too, and I prayed that he wouldn't. Luckily, he gave no sign that he remembered me. He was still the sweet, bashful guy I knew from grade school. According to the chart, he would stop taking his medication and end up in our emergency room, be admitted to the hospital to get stabilized, and then go back home. But even at his best, JB was unable to cope with school or work. He lived with his parents and never had a job or even a girlfriend, as far as I could tell.

I don't think JB ever remembered me from one hospital visit to the next. I'd see him in the ER and go out to say hi, and each time it was the same. We'd chat for a bit, there in front of the nurses station, and then he'd get this look on his face as if he was deciding whether he could trust me. It seemed he always decided he could, because next he would fish deep in the pocket of his jeans and pull out a worn sheet of paper, folded over and fuzzy at the edges. With a look of deep mystery and pride, he would unfold the paper and show me the picture. It was a motorcycle, detailed and beautifully drawn, with each part labeled—headlight, gearshift, tires. . . .

He told me it was his plan for the motorcycle he was building. He had no background in auto mechanics or motorcycle maintenance. According to his medical chart, he'd left school after twelfth grade and never worked. He spent his days wandering the neighborhood, sometimes dressed as a priest. Sometimes he mumbled blessings as he walked along. It was tragically clear that he lived entirely in his own imaginary world, unable to make the jump into the real world around him. I liked him so much that it was painful to realize he was as sick and disabled by schizophrenia as the many others I was seeing.

I always thanked him for sharing his drawing with me. Then he would fold it up and put it safely back in his pocket. It left me overwhelmed with sadness.

CHAPTER 3

The System Crashes

EATING FROM GARBAGE CANS: ROBBIE

On 2N, we psychiatry residents spent hours each day on discharge planning. Right after rounds, the three of us sat at the phone tables in the back of the ward and worked our way down the long list of board and care homes, calling and pleading until we found an opening. If you had a voluntary patient who was in no hurry to leave, you couldn't discharge them till they had a place to go.

We were always under pressure to open up beds. I didn't realize how great the pressure was until one afternoon when we discussed Robbie during team meeting. Robbie was a 19-year-old we were holding on a 14-day certification as gravely disabled. He was diagnosed with acute paranoid schizophrenia.

Robbie heard voices warning him that his parents were trying to kill him. He refused to go into the family home and was sleeping in his parents' garage. During the daytime he foraged in the neighbors' garbage cans for food. His frantic parents begged him to come inside but he refused. They took meals to him in the garage but he wouldn't touch anything from them.

During staff meeting we argued about what to do for Robbie. I campaigned along with the other interns to continue treating him while we could. But we were overruled. He was living in his parents' garage: he had shelter. He found his meals in garbage cans: he had food. Therefore he was not gravely disabled. Robbie was discharged that day.

Later I realized this was the harbinger of things to come, when hospital beds were so scarce that people like Robbie were considered not sick enough to warrant even a short stay in the hospital. And that hundreds, then thousands of others like Robbie would come to live on the streets, too frightened to stay in their family homes and scrounging through garbage cans for food.

HIGHLAND HOSPITAL

In 1983, I went to work as a staff psychiatrist at Highland Hospital in Oakland, which was the Alameda County hospital providing psychiatric care at that time. Since then, psychiatric hospital services have been transferred to John George Hospital in San Leandro, across the city line from Oakland.

When I started at Highland, I planned to stay for a long time. I thought it would be like Ward 2N at Chope Hospital, a gentle place where our patients usually stayed till they were better. But after a few weeks, my only goal was to work there long enough to buy a car. A small, inexpensive car.

Although the situation with Robbie at Chope was the exception, at Highland the extreme lack of beds made his experience the standard. Many of our patients at Highland were homeless, there for a respite from Hobo Park, an early homeless encampment in Oakland where they slept on the ground. But unlike at Chope, where we had to find a placement for each patient before discharge, at Highland, we simply wrote "Hobo Park" on the discharge papers and sent them out the door. I was dismayed.

I remember the first time I wrote "Hobo Park" on the discharge form. My patient was an old woman, and I was sending her back out to sleep on the ground again after her one day of hot meals and a warm bed in the hospital. She must have seen the look on my face because she leaned forward and patted my knee. "Don't worry," she said. "I have my own cardboard box in the park. It'll be there for me when I get back."

The ward was crowded with patients and staff, and we had no interview rooms. It was impossible to find a quiet spot where we could talk with our patients in private. But nobody seemed to think this was necessary, neither the staff nor the patients. It was a radical change from Ward 2N.

Our patients were sicker than at Chope, yet we gave them far less time than we'd given our patients there. Nearly all of them were on 5150s, but we rarely kept them for the full 72 hours. Beds were so scarce and the pressure to free them up so great that we sent people back out as soon as we could justify breaking their holds.

What we looked for was something we could document: a statement from the patient that today, as opposed to yesterday, he no longer intended to kill himself—or his wife, or his mother, or whoever had been the intended victim the day before. Then we could quote the patient's words and write, "not a danger to self or others." He didn't have to be convincing; he just had to say the right words, and then he was no longer "holdable."

So when we took our breaks, we staff psychiatrists limited our conversation to safe topics, like our mortgages. It was the first time I'd ever worked in a medical setting where my colleagues had no interest in talking about patients. We couldn't bear to think deeply about what we were doing.

Today it's common to read that physicians suffer from burnout. But one doctor suggested what we suffer from is "moral hazard." This term refers to profiting personally from an activity in which others take all the risk. Highland felt to me like a perfect example. After a year I'd leave with the money to buy a car, but my patients assumed all the risk: I would send them back out when they were still acutely psychotic, and I'd go home to my family.

What I remember today about Highland are the exceptions to this sad situation. One of my patients, a young drummer named Jack, had written to his girlfriend and told her he planned to kill her and cut her body into little pieces. In the letter he added grisly details about what he'd do with the pieces. Jack had a history of bipolar disorder and alcohol abuse and was amid a full-blown manic episode. I'd petitioned for a 14-day certification so we could treat him for two weeks longer.

I knew that Jack would most likely remain in this state of mind for more than two weeks, because manic episodes generally take longer than two weeks to resolve. And I knew that after the 14-day certification ended and he left the hospital, he would stop his medication. People in this state of mind have great difficulty believing that they need medication. I can understand why. The early phase of a manic episode creates a feeling of extreme well-being, soaring confidence, and boundless energy. You can go without sleep for long periods and feel uninhibited about approaching others, sure of your charm, and the rightness of your cause. For me, their booming confidence and high spirits are contagious.

But sometimes this phase can tip into an acute manic state. The tone of feeling changes from expansive well-being to irritability and impatience. A normally easygoing person can become quick to anger, even to violence, and pose a danger to the people around them.

They can endanger themselves, as well, due to their feeling of omnipotence, a grandiose belief in limitless power. This can lead to calamitous actions, such as jumping from a high place in the belief they can fly.

Jack had a history of high functioning and brilliant success as a drummer. He'd formed his own band, which played regular gigs, enough so that he supported himself with his music career. I was impressed. But occasionally this string of successes was broken by periods of illness, and he had a history of alcohol abuse.

At this point, Jack's life had already unraveled. He'd been thrown out of his own band. His words poured out in a furious jumble as he recounted how another drummer, a "mediocre hack," had taken his place. I knew he needed more treatment, but our hands were tied, as usual. As soon as he said he didn't plan to kill his girlfriend, we'd have to discharge him.

Even with all that had happened to him, Jack was engaging and self-assured. I assumed he would stop his lithium as soon as he left the hospital and instead use alcohol in a fruitless attempt to sleep and calm his nerves.

Then an amazing thing happened. The head of the psychiatry department came to the ward to talk to me about Jack. It turned out that his girlfriend's parents had extraordinary political leverage. They wanted action to protect their daughter, and the hospital couldn't ignore their demand.

Commitment for psychiatric observation and treatment is governed in California by the Lanterman-Petris-Short (LPS) law, a groundbreaking civil rights bill passed in 1967. This is the law that provides for the 72-hour hold if a patient is judged a danger to others or self or gravely disabled due to a mental disorder. A 14-day certification can extend the hold for another two weeks on the same basis, although due to our extreme shortage of beds, few patients actually stay in the hospital for this long. A second 14-day certification is possible (although extremely rare) if the patient can still qualify as a "danger to self." But after these two legal holds run out, it requires a conservatorship to extend the hold.

LPS law in California provides for commitment to a mental hospital for up to 90 days under extraordinary circumstances if the patient can be shown to be a danger to others due to a mental disorder. This extraordinary move requires an LPS conservatorship, with a conservator from the county public guardian's office overseeing the placement of the patient. The patient has the right to contest this commitment with a full jury trial. So we had a trial. I was in the strange position of teaming up with the district attorney to help him make his case for sending my patient to Napa, a nearby state hospital.

"Explain to the jury why we're here," said the public defender. "This young man looks perfectly normal." Jack did look very good. His beautiful shoulder-length hair was brushed and clean, he wore a dark blue suit, and his manner was irreproachable.

"He's on lithium," I said. "It's like having an umbrella. It's raining but the umbrella keeps you dry. The lithium is like an umbrella for the mind." Luckily there were many other witnesses, not just me. The jury found that he did indeed pose a danger to others due to his acute manic episode and needed to stay on his medication long enough to get through this episode. They found that he qualified for the 90-day commitment, and Jack went on to spend time at Napa Hospital, although far less than the full 90 days. At Highland we followed his progress through word of mouth. I was relieved to hear that he came home, his usual self again, rejoined his band, and broke up with his girlfriend without threats of violence.

The most successful patient I treated at Highland was John, a 25-year-old Hmong man who was profoundly depressed and had suicide plans. He was so quiet and so small and thin that he almost disappeared on that ward. When I tried to draw him out, he spoke in monosyllables, head down as if to hide from my prying eyes.

His people had strong family bonds and a deep belief in their own methods of healing. The Friday after John was admitted, his uncle came to visit and asked me if John could have a pass over the weekend. The family was conducting a healing ceremony for him.

I felt horribly torn. John needed the healing ceremony, I knew. He needed all the magic his people could create. He also needed to stay in the hospital for another week at least. I trusted that this caring family would watch over him and keep him safe through the weekend, but if I gave him a pass, he would lose his bed entirely. I felt terrible refusing.

"That's all right," said his uncle. "We can just use his jacket."

So he took his nephew's old black windbreaker, and they held the healing ceremony. John's uncle made a deep impression on me. He came to the hospital. He even managed to come to the ward. I imagined the gathering of relatives and the healing ceremony. John had a place in the world.

After another week, he was well enough to go home. That was an unusual outcome at Highland. I think his recovery was partly the anti-depressants. Certainly the healing ceremony helped. It was grounded in his native culture and must have been powerful for him. And most of all, John had his large family waiting for him. They were actively involved in his care. He belonged to his family, and they wanted him back.

SIDEWALKS AND JAILS REPLACE HOSPITALS

When Robbie, our young patient at Chope Hospital in San Mateo, believed his parents were trying to poison him and foraged in the neighbors' garbage for his meals and was judged no longer in need of treatment since he was able to survive on garbage, I was shocked. It was so callous, such a breach of our usual standard of care. But after a year at Highland, I knew Robbie's experience was not out of the ordinary; it was the usual state of care in California. Chope had been the aberration.

What I didn't know was why things were so bad. Then I learned about deinstitutionalization.

In the 1960s, American mental hospitals began to close their doors, first the large state hospitals and then the small community hospitals as well. By 1994, nearly half a million former patients had been sent back to live with their families. Often their families were unable to care for them, and the newly discharged patients ended up on the streets or behind bars. In Massachusetts, 27% of the newly discharged patients became homeless after six months. In Ohio, that figure was 36%, and in New York it was 38% (Torrey, 2012; 126).

And as hospitals closed down, the prison population skyrocketed. In 1960, 535,540 people were hospitalized for serious mental illness. By 2014, that number had fallen to 62,532 and is still falling. In 1960, 55,362 people with serious mental illness were behind bars. By 2014, that number had risen to 392,037 (Jaffe, 2017; 81, 187). So many former patients have been incarcerated that jails and prisons have become our de facto mental hospitals. Today, 90% of all inpatient psychiatric care in America is provided behind bars.

In the beginning, the hospital closure began naturally, when the first antipsychotic drugs were introduced in 1955. But then in 1965, the deinstitutionalization movement exploded, and the number of beds plummeted to a tenth of what they'd been forty years earlier. Behind this move was a political alliance of the far right and the far left.

On the political right were fiscal conservatives whose goal was to save money. In 1965, the federal government abruptly withdrew its financial support for the state hospitals, as well as the small community hospitals providing psychiatric care. This was accomplished by a little-known law, the Medicaid IMD Exclusion, passed by Congress in 1965 along with the creation of Medicaid (Jaffe, 2017; 82, 147). The IMD Exclusion forbids the use of Medicaid dollars to pay for care in a mental hospital. This left the states and counties responsible for the entire expense. It wasn't just the large state hospitals that were affected; any psychiatric hospital with more than 16 beds is forbidden to take Medicaid. Residential treatment facilities for chemical dependency were also forbidden to take Medicaid for patients over 21. After that, patients could use Medicare, but they had to wait until they were 65. In the meantime, only the very young, the very old, and the very well-financed can receive addiction treatment in a residential facility.

Psychiatric hospitals can still take private insurance, but due to the disabling effects of untreated mental illness, those who lack adequate treatment are often unable to work. Thus, they lack private insurance and are completely dependent on Medicaid. Medicaid is crucial to the survival of any hospital that serves the public and accepts patients without private insurance. Hospital treatment for severe mental illness can mean the difference between life and death, but because of this law, such treatment is specifically denied to the people who need it most. No other severe illness is subject to such discrimination.

Theoretically, the money saved would go toward community mental health care. This was the new mental health program proposed by President Kennedy as a replacement for the shuttered state hospitals (Jaffe, 2017; 185). But few of the taxpayers on the right or the left followed up on this plan, and community mental health was rarely funded. (San Mateo County has been one of the exceptions, maintaining something more akin to a real community mental health program.) We have come full circle from the early 19th century, when Dorothea Dix campaigned to rescue the insane from the prisons where they languished, often under shockingly inhumane conditions (Insel 2022; 25, 84). Due to her work, people with mental illness were rescued from prisons to be cared for in hospitals. But today that trend has been reversed. Once again, Americans with serious mental illness are being warehoused out of sight in our prisons.

ON THE LEFT: SZASZ, KESEY, AND REVOLUTIONARY ZEAL

The political Left worked along with the political Right to abolish hospital care for mental illness. In 1969, as a sophomore at Berkeley, I moved into Barrington Hall, where I heard much enthusiasm for this move. Barrington was a large student co-op just off Telegraph Avenue on the gritty south side of campus. We always had a small population of homeless people living with us in our large house. But there was a sense that the "street people," as we called them, were part of the revolution—they were nonconformists, our comrades in arms, even more oppressed than we were. We wanted to revolutionize a repressive society. The former hospitals symbolized that repression.

Often, I heard this refrain: "Mentally ill people are no more dangerous than anyone else. In fact, they're less apt to commit acts of violence." I took it as an indirect commentary on our discomfort with the street people who lived with us. And an acknowledgment that many of the street people had been patients in the newly shuttered state hospitals. People were afraid of them. I thought of my father, his violent rages, and his threats to start shooting. Of course, I kept these thoughts to myself.

Later studies showed that people released from the state hospitals were no more likely to commit acts of violence than others as long as they stayed on their medication or unless they also had problems with drugs. And if they did commit violent acts, these were mostly directed at their own family members, usually their parents and children. Torrey and Jaffe have written extensively about this issue (Torrey 2012, 148–52, 206–7; Jaffe 2017, 37).

In 1961, Thomas Szasz published *The Myth of Mental Illness* (1961), and on the left it was fashionable to argue that mental illness *was* a myth: what looked like insanity was actually the sane response to an insane society. With the war in Vietnam and our friends being sent off to fight in that crazy war, "society" could indeed seem insane.

While Szasz exerted wide influence over students and their professors, Ken Kesey spoke to the masses. *One Flew over the Cuckoo's Nest* came out in 1975 and swept the Academy Awards that year. The movie was based on his breakout novel by the same name, published in 1962.

The movie based on his book became a cultural touchstone, with lasting influence on the public. Today, almost 50 years after it came out, its shocking scenes are imprinted on the public consciousness. Many of us believe that this is what life is like in a psychiatric hospital. It's hard to unwind that belief and see the movie for what it was—a highly entertaining horror story with an antiestablishment rebel to root for.

As Kesey explains in his preamble to the novel, his first experience of a psych ward was as a subject in the early LSD experiments at Stanford

University. Every Tuesday for six months, he writes, he took his experimental dose, then spent the day in a small locked room with a window looking out onto the ward. Later he worked at that same hospital (the Menlo Park VA) as a nurses' aide on the night shift. At the time, Kesey was a graduate student at the Stanford writing program, and his experiences at that hospital gave him the material for his novel.

Even if he might have doubted some of the stories he heard, he had a gold mine of an opportunity to let his imagination—turbocharged on LSD—dream up terrifying scenes of abuse.

In his book, Kesey's narrator is "Chief" Bromden, a man overrun with psychotic delusions. Kesey carefully demonstrates Bromden's delusional state in the early pages of his book, signaling that Bromden is an unreliable narrator. In the book we see (through Bromden's eyes) Nurse Ratchet's arms elongate until they reach all the way across the ward and then wrap around hapless Black boys like a coiled rope. In Bromden's words, "she blows up bigger and bigger, big as a tractor, so big I can smell the machinery inside the way you smell a motor pulling too big a load" (Kesey, 1962; 5). In his mind, Big Nurse is not human but a monster robot.

But in the movie, the events that the delusional Bromden narrates in the book are shown as reality. The audience has no reason to doubt what they see on the screen—a lurid horror story presented as reality, with a cruelty hard to forget. As Ronald Reagan worked to shut down our psychiatric hospitals, the movie version of *Cuckoo's Nest* provided him with the perfect cover.

My experience working in such hospitals differs from the movie version. Although I worked at a half dozen psychiatric hospitals, one in Pittsburgh, Pennsylvania, and several in San Francisco and its suburbs, I can't remember seeing cruel treatment of patients by the staff. Instead, I saw overcrowding and the inability to admit people due to lack of beds and far too hasty discharge of patients who were still acutely ill, again due to lack of beds.

Many of our hospitalized patients were there on voluntary status. They came of their own volition and stayed as long as we could let them. This was especially true for patients who'd been on our inpatient service before—they knew what to expect and came back of their own accord. Often, Ward 2N was where they had first experienced real help with their psychotic illness.

I did see one incident of violence, which occurred at Highland. The victim was a nurse, and the assailant was a patient. A few of us were standing around the nurses station, talking, when a male patient came up to us and blindsided the nurse, punching him in the side of the head and knocking him to the floor. It came out of the blue. The nurse was a young man, gentle and unfailingly kind.

The Menlo Park VA Hospital, where Kesey took LSD and later worked, was certainly not the barbarous place depicted in the movie. It was and is a teaching hospital staffed by top-notch doctors and nurses. No nurse could have gotten away with the sadistic reign of terror Big Nurse visits on her defenseless patients. She would have lost her job if she treated her patients as she does in the group therapy scenes.

Nevertheless, we hear today that mental hospitals were "snake pits," based on the title of a 1948 movie starring Olivia de Havilland. Her character is truly psychotic but spends time in the hospital and is treated by a sympathetic and helpful psychiatrist. He is so kind to her that one of the nurses on the ward becomes jealous and arranges for her to be transferred to the "snake pit," a basement ward where the sickest patients are confined. She stays briefly until rescued by her kindly doctor.

King of Hearts, a French film that came out in 1966, gained cult status when I was a student in Berkeley. It contrasted the sane and cheerful inmates of the lunatic asylum with the war-weary townspeople, who flee because of a bomb scare, opening the asylum doors as they leave. It seemed to assure us that the people leaving the state hospitals and settling on our streets were indeed as sane as we were, perhaps more so. And that insanity was indeed a myth.

King of Hearts and *The Snake Pit* have largely faded from public awareness, but I believe the lesson of *Cuckoo's Nest* remains carved into our collective psyche. Since mental hospitals have always operated behind closed doors for reasons of confidentiality, there is no easy way to counter such dogma. Those of us who see mental illness up close—in our families, our patients, or even ourselves—might quietly chafe at this myth, but which of us is going to stand up and declare that we know mental illness is real, through a lifetime of experience? Or casually discuss our patients? We keep our mouths shut.

PEOPLE WRONGLY HOSPITALIZED

In 1973, American psychologist David Rosenhan published an influential paper, "On Being Sane in Insane Places," in *Science*, America's most prestigious scientific journal (Rosenhan, 1973). It landed, as *Cuckoo's Nest* had done, at a moment when the public was eager to hear his message. The paper purported to show that perfectly normal, healthy people were indiscriminately locked up in psychiatric hospitals by psychiatrists who wrongly labeled them as mentally ill. Since then, his paper has been widely cited. I remember it from my psychology classes in college.

The idea came to him as he sat in a lecture given by R. D. Laing, the popular and influential antipsychiatry psychiatrist from Scotland. Rosenhan reported that he used a ruse to support his claims. He wrote that he assembled a group of coconspirators and coached them on how to mimic acute psychosis. He gave them background stories that would make their acute psychotic episodes believable to an unsuspecting intake worker, he said, and sent them off. He reported that all eight of his accomplices gained admission to their assigned hospitals and then had trouble leaving the hospital.

Unlike other peer-reviewed medical or scientific studies, Rosenhan didn't include a methods and materials section to allow his readers to confirm the validity of his conclusions for themselves. Crucially, he never identified the hospitals or revealed the fake names his accomplices used. Regardless of this deficiency, his study made him instantly famous and was cited often as proof that psychiatric diagnosis is a sham and psychiatric hospitalization an outrage that should be abolished.

The fact that it was published in the prestigious journal *Science* without including the usual methods and materials section says much about the antipsychiatry climate of the times (Lieberman, 2023; 98–104). Lieberman attributes this profound hostility to psychiatry's embrace of psychoanalysis for much too long and without the scientific evidence to support it.

Although Rosenhan wrote that people with no mental illness easily fooled the psychiatrists, gained admission to eight different hospitals, and then were kept against their will, my experience has been the opposite. Often people try to gain admission to these hospitals, but the difficulty they have is getting in and staying in, not getting out.

In 1977, four years after Rosenhan's paper was published, I was on call, covering the emergency room at Chope Hospital. Already, even in prosperous San Mateo County, we had people who had lost their homes and were sleeping unsheltered. Many were army veterans, returned from Vietnam.

I remember one man who came to the ER at 3:00 a.m. I greeted him in the waiting room, brought him back to the exam room, and asked him what brought him to the ER that night. He blinked in the strong light. His eyes were red rimmed and his army jacket was mud stained and hung on his thin body.

"I'm hearing voices and feeling suicidal," he said. His eyelids drooped and then he fell asleep.

"Can you tell me more? Like, what's going on that you're wanting to hurt yourself?"

His head jerked up, and he looked at me in confusion. "What?"

"What's going on that you want to kill yourself?" I felt bad pressing him when it was so clear that what he needed was a warm bed.

"I'm hearing voices and feeling suicidal." Again he closed his eyes and slumped in his chair.

I was struggling to stay awake myself. "What are the voices saying?"

"Hmm? . . . I'm hearing voices and feeling suicidal."

I had heard this same phrase many times by then. I pictured the rumor passed around in homeless camps among disabled vets desperate for shelter: *Just say you're hearing voices and feeling suicidal. They'll put you in the psych ward.*

"Where are you staying right now?" I asked, feeling rotten for asking.

He looked at me with new attention. "In the park back there," he said, nodding in the direction of what I guessed was a patch of trees and grass. We didn't have any parks nearby.

"I'm so sorry, but I can't admit you to the hospital tonight. If you come back in the morning, you could talk to the social worker—"

He stood abruptly, his face full of pain and rage, and walked out into the night. I never saw him again.

Sometimes it was more complicated. Veronica was 31 years old and glamorous, with wide hazel eyes and a curtain of auburn hair. She repeatedly came to the Chope Hospital ER with the same complaint. She wanted to kill herself, she said, and would do so if not stopped. She had a plan—a bottle of Valium and a pint of Old Crow would do it, she said. *It certainly would*, I thought.

She was quietly furious, fuming under a facade of reasonability. Her boyfriend was treating her badly, she said. I didn't doubt that she was a threat to her own safety and told her we needed to hospitalize her for a couple days, till she was herself again.

At that she exploded with rage. "You people! I need care, and you put me in prison! Evil Nurse Ratched up there will force me to take drugs to *make* me sick. I'm not crazy, I'm sad."

I wanted to point out that no one would force medication on her unless she became violent and out of control, but I knew that would make her even more angry.

"I'm sorry," I said. "I'm afraid you might do what you say you're going to do, and then it will be too late."

She shot to her feet and glared at me, her face pale. "How do you know? You're not me."

"You're right. I don't know. I just have to make my best guess," I said.

"I hate you all," she said and turned away, studying the floor. I was afraid she was crying and suddenly I felt sad for her.

"Come on, I'll take you up," I said. "I just need to call ahead, make sure we have a bed for you."

She sank into the chair again, her face in her hands, while I called upstairs. I reached Suki, the nighttime charge nurse.

"Yes," she said, "we have beds."

As we rode up on the elevator, Veronica stared ahead, her face inscrutable. Suki met us at the door to the ward. She knew Veronica well from her many previous admissions and spoke to her in a soothing murmur.

In spite of our rocky beginning, I discovered the next day that Veronica would be my patient on the ward. I asked her if we could talk some more, and she exploded with a litany of charges—we were jailers, we treated her like a prisoner, we were incompetents who had no business locking her up. She was stiff with pride, and I tried not to crack her fragile veneer. I had written a 5150 that allowed us to keep her for up to 72 hours on the basis of danger to self, but when I tried to explain, she waved me away.

"I know all that shit," she said. She refused to talk with me any longer.

Later, when I looked at her chart, I saw she'd been hospitalized many times before on Ward 2N, with the same complaint: suicidal intent with a definite plan and the means to carry it out. Once she had called 911 and threatened to swallow the bottle of Valium as well as the half-pint of whiskey but then hung up. The 911 operator traced the call to her home and a couple of police officers checked on her. They knocked and rang, called to her through the door, explaining their reason for being there, but received no response. Alarmed and afraid she'd already carried out her threat, they tried the door but it was locked. In desperation, they broke down the front door and found her sitting calmly in the living room, watching as they struggled into the house to rescue her.

Veronica didn't seem psychotic. She was furious but always coherent. I never got that confused, blurry sensation that I sometimes experienced when I tried to follow the thread with our thought-disordered patients who suffered with schizophrenia. Previous doctors had given her a diagnosis of borderline personality disorder, which is not a major mental illness.

When I came to work the second morning, she was waiting for me as I let myself onto the ward. "My boyfriend's coming to take me home this morning." She had a glint of triumph in her eyes and looked nothing like the fragile woman I'd seen the day before. "I *hope* you're not planning to hold me."

"That's great," I said. "I just need to talk with you."

She followed me wordlessly and answered all my questions flatly. I could see she didn't need to be in the hospital, but I needed to hear in her own words that she was safe and document her statement in the chart, showing that I'd done another assessment and found her no longer a danger to herself. In those days, we kept accurate medical records and were accountable for our decisions.

Several weeks later, I was on call again when she came back to the ER and threatened suicide with the same plan. As before, she berated me for all the torture we inflicted on her by locking her up. We were jailers, not healers.

I have to confess, it annoyed me. "You know the system," I said. "You pull the levers of the system and then it does what it always does."

She was smart, and I could see that she understood what I was saying. I said it more in self-defense than to call her on her actions, and I didn't expect anything to change. But that was the last time she ended up on Ward 2N.

Five years later, I was working as a staff psychiatrist at Highland Hospital on one of its two psych wards. As soon as beds were vacated, we filled them with patients who'd been waiting downstairs in the ER to be admitted. We discharged patients as soon as we could write that they were no longer a danger to self or others in their chart note, which became part of their medical record. Most of our patients suffered from some form of severe mental illness—schizophrenia, most often, but sometimes bipolar disorder or major depression with suicidal intent.

In the midst of this sad chaos, I had one patient who didn't fit. He was a young man with tattoos on his arms—a skull and something that looked like graffiti. He was easy to talk to and held my gaze as he spoke of his deep desire to kill himself. He assured me that he had a powerful gun at home and would shoot himself in the head if I sent him out of the hospital. By then I'd seen many people who were contemplating suicide, and he showed none of the despair I'd come to expect, only a rigid attentiveness. As soon as I acknowledged his threat and assured him that we would keep him safe in the hospital, he seemed to relax.

When I saw him the next day, his mood was buoyant. "You can keep me for three days on this 5150, right? And then if I'm still suicidal, you can put me on two 14-day holds, so I might be in here for a month. Right?"

"I could but that would be extraordinary," I said. "I've never had anyone in this hospital for more than a week."

His exultant mood seemed to collapse.

"But let's talk about what's making you so unhappy."

"I just am," he said, not meeting my eyes now.

"What's going on?" I asked.

He didn't answer for a long time. Instead he turned his face away from me, and I saw him wipe tears.

"Oh, goodness," I said. "Please—tell me what's going on."

He paused even longer, staring down into his lap and clenching his hands. Finally he said, "I'm not safe out there. There's people who want to kill me."

With that, I saw him in a new light. "You're not in a gang, are you?"

He shrugged, still not looking at me. "Maybe."

I liked him and of course I didn't want anything to happen to him. But I couldn't give him one of our precious beds for the next month, when dozens of others really needed that bed. "Maybe we could find somewhere safe, somewhere besides the hospital."

In the end we arranged for his brother to come to the ward and escort him to safety. My patient would stay with his grandmother, who'd known nothing about this side of his life until that moment.

More than 30 years after Rosenhan published his paper in *Science*, Susannah Cahalan, who wrote *Brain on Fire: My Month of Madness* (2012) about her own experience as a patient in a mental hospital, reviewed his study. She examined the documents left behind by him after his death and published her findings in *The Great Pretender* (Cahalan, 2019). Here she questioned the veracity and validity of the Rosenhan experiment. Based on her examination of those documents, Cahalan reported apparent distortion in the *Science* article. She cited inconsistent data, misleading descriptions, and inaccurate or fabricated quotations from psychiatric records. Moreover, despite an extensive search, she was able to identify only two of the eight pseudo patients: Rosenhan himself and a graduate student whose testimony is allegedly inconsistent with Rosenhan's description in the article.

In light of these findings, Cahalan questioned whether some or all of the six other pseudo patients might have been simply invented by Rosenhan. A few years later, Andrew Scull of the University of California at San Diego wrote "Rosenhan Revisited: Successful Scientific Fraud," in which he agreed with Cahalan's conclusions. He published his article in the peer-reviewed journal *History of Psychiatry* (Scull, 2023).

Despite this indication of fabrication in Rosenhan's work, it continues to be cited to this day. Few people know who Cahalan and Scull are, and their work is virtually unknown. What remains are Rosenhan's claims, which, 50 years later, still influence our debate about how best to help those stricken with severe mental illness.

CHAPTER 4

Economic Causes of Homelessness

PANHANDLING FOR A LIVING: KYLE

Homelessness as we know it today is a new phenomenon. Fifty years ago, Americans did not live on the streets in the way they do today. Waves of homelessness occurred during economic cataclysms, such as the Panic of 1873 and the Great Depression. But when those hard times ended, the unemployed found work and shelter. Policies initiated in the '60s and '70s created a new brand of homelessness—a deeply marginalized population who live on the streets even in times of general prosperity.

In 2016 I set out to interview people living on the streets. I wanted to know how they had ended up there, who they were, and how they survived. It felt a bit intrusive to approach people and ask them for interviews. True, they were living in full view of the public, but still, that patch of sidewalk was their living room. Then I met Kyle.

Kyle had a spot on Telegraph Avenue, a few blocks south of the UC Berkeley campus, with a cardboard sign that read, "Just need weed." He flashed me a winning smile as I approached and said, "But money will do." He agreed to share his story with me, and I joined him, cross-legged on the pavement, with my phone set between us to record the interview. He told me he'd been living on the streets for twenty years, ever since he turned eighteen and left his foster family. As far as he knew, his own family was still in Arizona, but he had lost track of them long ago.

A cold wind blew off the bay, and Kyle was wrapped in a pale yellow blanket smudged with dirt. Under that, he wore an oversized army surplus jacket with the hood up. Only his hands and face were exposed to the frigid air. He was missing all his lower teeth on one side, as if at some point he'd taken a calamitous punch in the mouth. His fingers bore crude tattoos, and the ground-in dirt covered him like an extra layer of skin.

Kyle couldn't remember the year he should have graduated from high school, or even which decade that would have been. But when he turned eighteen, he aged out of foster care and suddenly he was on his own without a job. "So how did you support yourself all these years?" I asked. He nodded at the upturned hat on the sidewalk in front of him. It held one quarter.

Kyle claimed he was living well in Berkeley. "Every Saturday morning they feed all the people in the park so I usually hang out and get tons of food." Although he claimed to eat "all the time," Kyle was bone thin.

"Where will you sleep tonight?" I asked.

His expression turned wary. "I usually pick random spots—makes it safer. Like, this is chill, you know, and I just go there."

"Not a homeless shelter?"

"Nah—you get most of the crazies there." He grimaced. "It always smells like feet—and I wake up with my stuff stolen." With that, he straightened up and looked me in the eye. "It's a scientifically proven fact," he said, "that anyone on the street has post-traumatic stress. And anyone who doesn't have it should be considered not right in the head. But I know how to roll with it."

A pair of young women in distressed blue jeans and soft leather boots appeared at this point, offering clean needles and condoms. Kyle waved them away. At first this seemed like a good sign. Perhaps it's true that he does "just need weed," I thought. But then his speech began to slur. His sentences stopped making sense. He had trouble keeping his head up, and I realized he was nodding off. Whatever he was using to "roll with it" was a lot stronger than weed.

LOSS OF OUR INDUSTRIAL BASE

Not so long ago, it would have been easy for an unskilled worker like Kyle to find a job to supply his basic needs. But things have changed. Since 1980, several million manufacturing jobs have been lost, mostly due to offshoring (Kimball and Scott, 2014). These had been good jobs with benefits, meaning workers could support families. And those families in turn supported local businesses and contributed to community life. But after being laid off, if the newly unemployed found work at all, it was usually temporary or part-time work. Millions of households fell into poverty.

The North American Free Trade Agreement (NAFTA) was passed in 1994, and in 2001 China was admitted to the World Trade Organization (WTO). President Clinton, who signed NAFTA into law and campaigned for China's admission to the WTO, assured the public that these free trade agreements would usher in a new age of American prosperity. China, in particular, would provide a vast new market for American-made goods (Clinton, 2000). Instead, American workers by the millions lost their jobs when production was moved to countries with cheaper labor.

In 2000, Robert Scott of the Economic Policy Institute (EPI) wrote that even by the administration's own analysis, "spiraling deficits and job losses" were predicted (Scott, 2000).

In 2013, David Autor and Gordon Hanson estimated that 2.5 million jobs had been lost to Chinese imports alone (Autor and Hanson, 2013).

Later, in "China Trade, Outsourcing and Jobs," Kimball and Scott of the EPI wrote that the "[g]rowing U.S. trade deficit with China cost 3.2 million jobs between 2001 and 2013, with job losses in every state." They estimated that 55% of the jobs lost between 2001 and 2013 were caused by offshoring to China (Kimball and Scott, 2014).

In "The Zombie Robot Argument Lurches On," Lawrence Mishel and Josh Bivens argued that although automation is frequently blamed for job loss, it has had minimal impact (Mishel and Bivens, 2017). *The Reshoring Initiative* echoes this conclusion. In a March 10, 2017, blog post, they write that 4.6 million manufacturing jobs have been lost to offshoring and recommend reshoring to restore our manufacturing base (Reshoring Initiative, 2017).

Deaths of Despair and the Opioid Crisis

The tragic epidemic of opioid addiction and overdose is in the news every day, and I won't repeat what's already well known. The Sacklers systematically and cynically carried out an advertising campaign to persuade doctors to prescribe OxyContin, urging them to ever-higher doses for an ever-growing list of complaints.

What receives less attention is the relevance of job loss to this epidemic and the effects of these mass layoffs due to offshoring. In 2015 two economists, Anne Case and Angus Deaton, spoke out about their research on what they termed "deaths of despair" from suicide, drug overdose, and alcoholism. What they noticed first was the startling increase in early deaths among white men during the past two decades. Examined more closely, it turned out that this change was driven by the rising death rate specifically among white men without a college education. That rise was so steep that it pulled the whole demographic up with it. Among white men with a college degree there was little change, as was the case for Black men.

Case and Deaton published their groundbreaking book, *Deaths of Despair and the Future of Capitalism*, after exhaustive research on the economic causes of this calamity. What they found was a sharp divide between the fortunes of Americans with a bachelor's degree and those with only a high school diploma, especially among white men. This makes sense, as the workers who had been laid off by the millions from their factory jobs were mostly white men with only a high school education. But those factory jobs had sustained them and even allowed them to flourish. The collapse of our manufacturing base created a wide employment gap. In 2017, 84% of Americans with a bachelor's degree or more were employed, whereas only 64% of those with just a high school diploma were employed (Case and Deaton, 2020).

It turns out that what's been happening to white working-class men during the last twenty years is a repeat of what happened three decades earlier in Black inner city communities. "The first wave of globalization hit blacks particularly hard, and jobs in the central city became scarce for this long-disadvantaged group" (Case and Deaton, 2020; 5). This massive job loss in the 1970s and 1980s devastated family and community life, and the situation worsened with an epidemic of crack cocaine and HIV, the latter spread by IV drug use. What followed was a sharp increase in mortality among Black men. "[D]ecades later, less educated whites, long protected by white privilege, were next in line" (Case and Deaton, 2020; 62). Today more than half of white working-class Americans believe that discrimination against whites has become as big a problem as discrimination against Blacks (Case and Deaton, 2020; 6).

"During that earlier episode of black despair, job loss, and family and community destruction," they write, much of the dysfunction was attributed to peculiarities of Black culture. Now this episode looks like something different, that if any group is treated badly enough for long enough, it is susceptible to suffering social breakdown of one kind or another" (Case and Deaton, 2020; 189).

Other ethnic groups have suffered increasing deaths of despair during the last two decades. Although the suicide rate has increased among all ethnic groups, Native Americans have suffered the most, far outpacing every other ethnic group by 2017 (Curtin and Hedegaard, 2019).

Whereas job loss and unemployment are generally seen as financial problems, amenable to such simple solutions as a universal basic income (UBI), these authors argue otherwise. "It is the loss of meaning, of dignity, of pride and of self-respect . . . the loss of marriage and community that brings on despair, not just or even primarily the loss of money" (Case and Deaton, 2020; 8).

Between 1995 and 2015, the death rate for white men aged 45 to 54 without a college degree tripled. And the younger the men, the higher their death rate. "The later you were born, the higher the risk of dying a death of despair at any given age," they note (Case and Deaton, 2020; 49–61).

Case and Deaton also address the effects of the meritocracy and the growing separation between the more and the less educated. This development has profound implications for American politics. The divide looks different depending on where you stand. Asked about the effects of college education on the country, those with less education thought it was having a negative effect.

The authors quote Michael Sandel on this point: "Winners are encouraged to consider their success their own doing—and to look down upon those less fortunate than themselves. Those who lose out may complain that the system is rigged, that the winners have cheated and manipulated their way to the top. Or they may harbor the demoralizing thought that their failure is their own doing, that they simply lack the talent and drive to succeed" (Sandel, 2018).

One result of this growing divide is that the wealthier, more educated and the poorer, less educated no longer live and work together. In *Glass House*, Brian Alexander makes this point about his own hometown of Lancaster, Ohio (Alexander, 2017). The Lancaster of his childhood was a thriving center of glass manufacture. Alexander went to school with the children of glass workers and the children of factory owners. The parents knew one another and rubbed elbows at school events. But then the factories were bought out, leveraged for investment elsewhere, and finally shut down and the contents sold off for scrap. The factory owners now lived far away, having no roots in Lancaster and no desire to live there. As those left behind lost their livelihoods, their children looked forward to a bankrupt future, and gradually the opioid epidemic manifested in Lancaster.

UNEMPLOYMENT FIGURES ARE UNAFFECTED

Despite the millions of jobs lost in manufacturing and the poverty that followed, our unemployment figures have remained excellent. The U.S. Bureau of Labor Statistics comes up with these figures based on household surveys (U.S. Bureau of Labor Statistics, n.d.). The official unemployment figure counts only Americans who are part of the "workforce," meaning those who are employed or currently looking for work (based on a job application in the last four weeks). Others, such as those who want to work but have given up looking for a job, are not counted. People living on the streets are seldom counted, as it is extremely difficult to apply for a job while living homeless. Receiving unemployment benefits is not an indication of being unemployed for the Bureau of Labor Statistics. Since these numbers are derived from household surveys, people living in single-room occupancy hotels, which house adults at the margins of society, are not counted. Those living behind bars are specifically excluded.

Meanwhile, as manufacturing shifted overseas, corporate profits skyrocketed while the wages of ordinary American workers, those who still had work, stagnated.

The outrageous truth is that people impoverished through lack of work don't count as unemployed. And any job, no matter how temporary or how few the hours, counts as employment. As a result of this specious method of calculation, the tectonic shift of industrial jobs away from the United States never registered as a rise in unemployment. In January 2020, the official unemployment rate was 3.6%.

HOUSING VANISHES AND THE SAFETY NET UNRAVELS

Meanwhile, one million units of low-cost housing were lost due to changes in public policy. Until 1974, federal programs such as Section 8 housing had provided direct assistance to low-income households. With a Section 8 voucher, an impoverished renter could secure an apartment because the federal government would cover most of the rent.

Then in 1974, President Ford signed into law the Housing and Community Development Act and everything changed. Funds that formerly supported Section 8 were given to the states as block grants to be administered as they saw fit, with no requirement to maintain the programs that formerly helped house the poor. The Section 8 program has withered for lack of funding, and the bulk of federal housing assistance has wound up in the pockets of property owners, largely through tax advantages. Urban renewal became the new priority for the Department of Housing and Urban Development (HUD). With generous funding through HUD, urban renewal destroyed much of the remaining housing available to the poor.

The city of Oakland provides a good example of urban renewal. In 1999, when Jerry Brown was elected mayor of Oakland, the city had been losing population. Brown promised to bring 10,000 new residents to the city, his "10K plan." Some residents cheered this plan (Avalos, 2015). Others criticized it for taking HUD funds meant for low-income housing and diverting them to the development of luxury apartments.

The downtown Oakland and Jack London Square neighborhoods were the priority.

Prior to the 10K plan, there were 24 residential hotels in downtown Oakland. These hotels, also known as single-room occupancy hotels (SROs), had always been the last refuge for the very poor. Brown planned to replace the SROs with market-rate and "affordable" housing. "Affordable" is a vague and relative term. One definition I've found is "no more than fifteen percent above the median price" of homes in the area. In 2023, that would mean that $862,500 for a house in Oakland qualifies as "affordable."

Terry Messman, writing for *Street Spirit* at the time, called Brown's plan a Trojan horse. "The hidden part of this so-called '10K' plan," he wrote, "is to drive away all the social problems and poor people that might make downtown Oakland an unappealing place to live for your average, upwardly mobile dot-commer." He challenged the mayor to respond to the poor residents who'd been squeezed out of their homes. "What is the plan, Mayor?" he wrote. "Where are the poorest residents of West Oakland supposed to go?" (Messman, 2016).

While low-cost housing was vanishing, safety-net programs such as Aid to Families with Dependent Children (AFDC) were being cut as well. In 1996, President Bill Clinton signed into law what was billed as welfare reform (Politico, 2018). Like HUD funding for Section 8, AFDC was replaced by block grants for the states to spend as they liked, with no guarantees of even minimal support for children and families in poverty.

The philosophy behind welfare reform was that welfare was bad for recipients because it fostered dependence. These beliefs were fueled by a deep anger among voters who imagined that they were being taken for a ride by Cadillac-driving welfare queens. Under the new law, families fell further into poverty, often losing their homes in the process. The deceptively low unemployment figures fed the belief that anyone who wanted to work could find a job.

Although people living on the streets are often assumed to be mentally ill, it turns out that only about one third of them are homeless due to mental illness. Job loss and destruction of housing and the social safety nets are responsible for two thirds of our homeless population.

Hoping for Shelter

In 2017, the Berkeley City Council planned to build lockers for homeless people so they could store their belongings safely. I was writing for the *East Bay Express* at the time, assigned to talk with people living on the streets and get their reactions to the proposal. None of them had heard of the plan, and when I explained it, they seemed puzzled. Where was it again? How would they get there?

So I gave up and asked what more they thought the city could be doing for them. One especially talkative young man lit up when I told him I was writing for the *East Bay Express.*

"Oh, yeah, I like that paper." He told me they got it at John George (the county mental hospital) and sometimes at Santa Rita (the county jail).

What else could the city do for people living on the street? He didn't hesitate. "More 5150s." He smiled. "I take lots of meth and go out on the streets, and pretty soon I'll get picked up." He paused and added, "I like John George better than Santa Rita."

I pictured him out on the street, wild with amphetamine psychosis, carried off by the police. Then, at John George or maybe Santa Rita, he'd get a clean bed and some regular food. A brief moment of respite from the cold sidewalk. Although some homeless people do take advantage of homeless shelters when beds are available and some manage to live in their cars or even in RVs parked on the street, this young man, like Kyle, was one of the many "street homeless."

Certainly there is a high incidence of drug use among people living on the streets, but it may be that drug abuse follows homelessness rather than the other way around. People take stimulants to stay awake at night and protect themselves from theft or physical attack. And like Kyle, people take drugs to cope with the stress, to "roll with it."

One writer for *Street Spirit* spelled out the traumatic sequence of events leading to street homelessness. First, he wrote, you lose your job. Then, as you struggle to find another job, you drain your bank account in an effort to pay the rent and hold onto your apartment. When your money runs out and you're evicted for nonpayment of rent, you couch surf for as long as your family and friends will have you. After their hospitality runs out, you move into your car. But it costs money to maintain your car, and eventually your car is towed. Then you pack all your belongings into one bundle and camp out on the sidewalk.

I've always been struck by this description of the descent into homelessness and the fact that it begins with job loss. Often our discussions of homelessness conclude with another call to build more housing, but I think it will take much more. We need to restore Section 8 by fully funding this program, and once more provide housing vouchers to the poor. We need to restore AFDC, so poor families with children can stay in their homes. We need to drastically reduce our use of prisons, as a history of incarceration often means a life sentence of joblessness. But most of all, we need to provide jobs for the millions of our people who have no work.

CHAPTER 5

Chemical Dependency

A Personal Foray into Addiction

As a sophomore at Berkeley, I moved to Barrington Hall, a huge student co-op where we always had a few "street people" living with us. One day I went up to our rooftop laundry room, which was occupied by a couple of men who were cooking heroin using a bottle cap and a cigarette lighter. They offered to share it with me.

I declined the offer. But I did take up smoking, fully planning to become addicted. In my future life as a social worker, I saw myself ministering to heroin addicts. To truly understand what they were facing, I thought, I should experience addiction for myself. Nothing prolonged, just a quick in and out. Also, I wanted to lose ten pounds.

We had a cigarette machine, of course, in the lobby at Barrington Hall, and one of my duties as the switchboard manager was to cart away last year's stale cigarettes after they'd been replaced with fresh stock. My plan was to smoke up those old cigarettes and then quit.

Five years later I was in Pittsburgh, starting medical school, still trying to stop smoking. The school had a snack bar on the ground floor with little Formica tables where we drank coffee between classes. There were ashtrays, too, for the smokers. It was just us students there except for Professor Melanie Graves, who sat and smoked with us in those first months. She was not much older than we were, a humble and quiet woman who always had a cigarette going. She was a pathologist and would be our pathology professor next year. I was dreading that course, knowing we'd be looking at lungs full of cancer. I'd be helplessly smoking, terrified of what it was doing to me.

One day I joined Dr. Graves at her little table. "You see cancerous lungs all the time," I said. "How can you keep smoking?"

She gave a long, sad sigh. "I'm always trying to quit, but then I get a frozen section from a patient with possible breast cancer. They put the surgery on hold while I look at the slides to determine if it's malignant or not. As soon as I get those slides, I reach for a cigarette."

I felt sorry for her and still more worried for myself. If Melanie Graves couldn't quit, with everything she saw, my own chances looked dismal. I woke up every morning planning to stop, and every night I'd be down at that corner store, buying another pack.

Then out of nowhere, my mother arranged for me and my sister Helen to spend a week together at our grandparents' cottage in Michigan. My mother and her family had spent summers there when she was a child. There was a rustic dining hall and docks along the lake with an assortment of canoes and sailboats. I figured if there was ever going to be a chance for me, that would be it. I planned to use that retreat as my own residential treatment program, a chance to be out of my usual environment and away from all pressure to perform.

The first thing I saw when we got to the cottage was a long, barely smoked cigarette lying in a large glass ashtray on the card table in the living room. I could rip the filter off (for sanitary reasons) and smoke the rest of it unfiltered.

That almost-whole cigarette burned a hole in my brain. You might think I'd throw it out just to make everything simple and safe. Instead, I stowed the ashtray on a high shelf in the pantry. Just in case.

Helen and I had the cottage to ourselves. We sailed on the lake, played cards, read our books, and talked. We saw just enough of the aunts and uncles and cousins to be appropriately sociable. By the end of the week, I'd eaten twenty-one meals at the dining hall without smoking a cigarette afterward. I'd drunk coffee every day without a cigarette to go with it. I retrieved the big glass ashtray from the pantry, threw away that disgusting cigarette butt, wiped out the ashtray, and put it back on the card table.

At school that fall, I bought my copy of Big Purple, our huge pathology textbook. I lugged it home with me and turned to the section on lung cancer. Amazingly, my chances of getting lung cancer from smoking were only 6%. All that struggle for 6%? I felt cheated.

On the other hand, Melanie Graves never came back to teach us. She had fallen into that 6% and died of lung cancer.

Heroin in the Haight

At the end of our second year, each of us medical students had to find an independent study project for the summer. It could be anything we chose, anywhere, as long as it was medical. Vaguely medical was okay. I'd gotten a clerkship in Erie, Pennsylvania, where I'd be trailing after a family practice doctor. Then I saw a posting for San Francisco: "Drug Abuse Training Program for Medical Students" at the Haight Ashbury Free Clinic. I knew that fleeing to California and spending a summer in the Haight wasn't going to advance my career in medicine. I told myself I should go to Erie, then I flew home to San Francisco.

The "Summer of Love" in San Francisco had ended eight years earlier and left behind an epidemic of heroin addiction. The Haight Ashbury Free Clinic cared for many of these addicts, and Daryl Inaba, the Free Clinic pharmacist, was our teacher for that summer program.

Daryl was the ideal person to fill that role. He had long hair, down to his shoulders, to signal that he was not as straight an arrow as we might think. On the other hand, he understood addiction and taught us the basics. "The definition of addiction," he said, "is compulsive drug use, with inability to stop in spite of adverse consequences." He repeated it like a mantra. I thought of my struggle to quit smoking, with the fear of lung cancer always lurking in my mind, how I had pushed it aside and told myself, "Just today."

Daryl knew how these drugs worked, a thing I was deeply curious about. He was the first person I heard who explained why crack was so addictive. "That white powder cocaine we all know," he said, "cook it with baking soda and you get crack, which doesn't break down at high temperatures, so you can smoke it. That is a huge advantage." This way, you can use the entire surface of your lungs to absorb it. And your lungs are perfectly designed for gas exchange.

"And crack is fat soluble, so it crosses the blood-brain barrier and goes straight into your brain. Instant high; over-the-moon high."

The blood-brain barrier allows fat-soluble substances into the brain more readily than water-soluble substances because of the large volume of white matter in the brain, with its high fat content. If the human body were a bottle of salad dressing, the brain would be the oily top layer and the rest would be the watery bottom layer.

We learned about the various methods of taking heroin, their advantages and disadvantages. IV injection leaves tracks, transmits disease, and risks pulmonary embolism when the drug is cut with talc. It also risks fatal overdose; because you inject it all at once, you can't gauge the dosage as you go along. Much better, Daryl explained, is to smoke it. You could use a pipe. Or you could burn a lump of raw heroin and inhale the smoke through a straw. "Chasing the dragon," he called it. He said it with a certain relish, as if he could see that little smoking dragon.

We had nothing but counseling to offer the crack users. But we had drugs to cope with heroin withdrawal: Darvon-N, which acted on the opiate receptors in the brain to stop the drug craving. Tylenol for pain, Bentyl for diarrhea, and Librium for anxiety. The Darvon-N was supposed to be tapered over six days—six the first day, five the second day, and so on till the heroin withdrawal ended. But often our clients took the first day's pills and never came back. Or, just as often, they'd make it through withdrawal and then relapse. Daryl said, "We give them drugs to bribe them into counseling."

I'm not sure the counseling did much good. I spent hours each day at the detox clinic, a drafty old Victorian house with many nooks and crannies, odd little rooms where we saw our clients. All of them were heroin addicts. But I found myself unexpectedly charmed by these hard-core drug users. One of my classmates in the program, a clean-cut guy from Oklahoma who worked at the detox clinic with me, expressed the same sense of wonder. "I just listened to that guy for an hour," he said. "I like him, and I want to see him back. Even though right now he's probably stealing the radio out of my car." He laughed at the irony.

At the end of summer, I went back to Pittsburgh, where we gathered in small groups to report on our projects. As I recounted my experiences treating heroin addicts in San Francisco, one of the faculty leaned over to the professor next to him and spoke loud enough for me to hear. "What a waste," he said. "Let 'em die."

I knew that addicts were pariahs. But his words only pushed me further in the direction I'd always been headed. Somehow, these outcasts were my people.

SOLDIERS BATTLE AT HOME

When I finished my residency, it wasn't much of a leap for me to sign on for a two-year physician fellowship in substance abuse treatment. It was at the Fort Miley VA Hospital in San Francisco. I thought it would be fun. Also, my husband and I had bought a house in west Berkeley, a fixer-upper that needed massive fixing up. For a while it was interesting, seeing what was inside the walls, which needed to be replaced, and discovering the mysteries of Sheetrock. But it consumed all our weekends, all our vacation time, and all our money. The VA fellowship paid $40,000 a year, a fabulous sum that would set us free.

The VA sponsored this fellowship because so many soldiers were coming home from Vietnam addicted to heroin and suffering from post-traumatic stress disorder (PTSD), and they couldn't find enough physicians trained in substance abuse treatment, especially among psychiatrists.

Again, I worked at the detox clinic and saw heroin addicts, but this time I saw them for ongoing therapy. I worked on the inpatient alcohol treatment unit and saw those patients for ongoing therapy as well.

I thought of the winters in Pittsburgh, when all the dead leaves and trash and rusty, abandoned tools disappeared under a thick cover of snow. It was breathtaking, miraculous to my California eyes. And then in the spring, all that trash and those rusty tools reappeared.

Drug addiction, I decided, was like that snow. The ongoing intoxication covered up everything underneath. I had a patient who came to the clinic complaining of severe depression, requesting antidepressants. I asked him to hold off on the alcohol, so we could see what he was like without it. Alcohol itself is a central nervous system (CNS) depressant, and with the alcohol out of his system, his sadness evaporated. Amazingly, for both of us.

But I learned that you have to wait for the snow to melt, so to speak. Another patient, an ex-major in the army and now an executive for an insurance firm, came for help with her compulsive drinking. She drank alone, when she was safely home. After starting our program, she was thoroughly disciplined about her recovery, attending the ninety meetings in ninety days that Alcoholics Anonymous (AA) advises. But after those three months, she found herself in a crushing depression. We wondered together if she'd been drinking to cover her depression, but we didn't wait to find out. She began a course of Elavil, a common antidepressant at that time, and finally she began to be interested in life. She went out at night with friends, and then she fell in love.

A young ex-marine I saw at the VA Detox Clinic was not as lucky. While he managed to get free of his heroin addiction, he still suffered from flashbacks and then hallucinations. He saw a severed head rolling away—the same head, over and over. When I left the VA, he was still suffering from that horrifying vision.

Another of my patients was an accountant, a partner in a large firm in the city. When he disappeared one day, his worried partners searched the city for him and finally located his car in the parking lot of a cheap motel. He'd retreated to that dismal place in order to drink without interruption. He was lucky to be found; a surprising number of suicides are preceded by just such a solitary binge.

He completed the VA's 28-day inpatient alcohol treatment program and went on to live in a halfway house for the next year, where he drove the van transporting the other residents to their 12-step meetings. It was important for him to have this period of safety, living in a halfway house, away from his usual life, with nothing more stressful to do than driving the van.

I understood how important this zone of safety was to his recovery, remembering that week in Michigan with my sister, away from all the pressures of my life at home. The long-term residential programs for people struggling with addiction work the same way. They provide an oasis of respite from the demands of regular life and away from the myriad cues that lead to cravings and drug hunger. In that zone of safety, you can endure the anxiety of not using the drug you depend on, and gradually that life without your drug becomes bearable, even comfortable.

My patient was steadfast in his recovery program, motivated not so much by his desire to get back to work, but to see his young daughter. His ex-wife had forbidden him to see her due to his alcohol use, but now she was allowing him brief visits. Each week he told me about those visits.

"I thought I'd never see her again, and when I holed up in that motel, I meant to die."

STRUGGLE AND RECOVERY: KAISER OAKLAND

In the 1980s, Oakland was swamped with crack cocaine. In 1984 I went to work at Kaiser Oakland, with a mandate to revamp their substance abuse program. When I arrived, it was staffed by a skeleton crew of two part-time nurse practitioners and one psychiatrist, who was leaving.

We got together, the nurses and I, and designed a new program. We stopped writing prescriptions for Valium and started groups. Groups for recovering alcoholics, groups for adult children of alcoholics (ACAs), and groups for recovering cocaine addicts. We ran evening clinics so people with jobs could come after work. We hired two psychologists, doubling the size of our staff.

We visited local 12-step meetings and compiled a list of the ones we liked to recommend for our patients. The 12-step programs included Alcoholics Anonymous (AA), Narcotics Anonymous (NA), Overeaters Anonymous (OA), Adult Children of Alcoholics (ACAs), and other similarly focused groups. I'd never been to an AA meeting, and it wasn't like what I'd seen in the movies. No one was put on the spot or even asked for his or her name. Instead I felt a sense of safety. There was a check-your-weapons-at-the-door feel to those meetings.

In our Kaiser groups, we cultivated the same spirit of intentional kindness. Our alcohol groups and our ACA group were lively and seemed to be helpful, often in ways that surprised me. One woman came to our alcohol group for months but never said a word. Then when we met privately, she told me the group had been enormously helpful. She had quit drinking and was staying sober. Up until that moment, I'd believed that if you didn't talk, you got nothing out of therapy. But it seemed that just sitting in that group and listening could be transformative.

People would stay in those groups for months, even years. Listening as they talked, I learned about HALT, one of the many AA aphorisms. It's a systematic reminder of all that might be going on with you when you're trying to stay sober and want a drink: ask yourself if you're hungry, angry, lonely, or tired. It captures an essential quality of alcohol addiction: coping skills deteriorate and self-awareness fades as every twinge of discomfort translates into the need for a drink.

We petitioned the Kaiser administration for a room where we could sponsor an AA group on-site and were given a meeting room in a far corner of the campus. I spoke to the slightly grumpy maintenance worker who'd been given the additional chore of setting up the room. He busied himself with the chairs until I explained our purpose and then he turned to me with a wide smile. "I'm in the program myself," he said. "Anything you need, just ask."

Our cocaine group was a different story. Cocaine withdrawal left people jumpy and angry, and we had little to offer them to combat that withdrawal. To this day, no one has found an effective drug to combat cocaine withdrawal.

Cocaine acts to flood the brain with dopamine. Large quantities of dopamine are released into the neural synapses, causing a feeling of extreme well-being, high energy, and boundless self-confidence. In the process, the dopamine storage vesicles at the ends of those transmitting neurons are depleted. After a run of cocaine use, there is too little dopamine left to maintain an even mood. During withdrawal, the brain is starved for dopamine, leaving the user unable to experience pleasure or hope. The only thing that relieves that misery is more cocaine, although as time goes on, it has less and less effect due to the shortage of dopamine in the transmitting neurons.

In our cocaine groups, people told of digging between the couch cushions for crumbs of crack cocaine and everybody nodded. They'd been there too. Till the advent of crack, these addicts had lived normal lives with families and jobs. They had no history of mental illness or substance abuse. Then they would smoke crack cocaine or freebase (crack in its purified form), usually at a party, with friends.

That first experience worked on their minds. They found themselves craving the drug in a way they'd never imagined. They didn't recognize themselves. Money flew out of their savings, husbands or wives left, houses were lost, and they moved in with their mothers. The last thing to go was always their employment. When their work suffered, their human resources managers referred them to us for treatment as a condition of keeping their jobs. The story was depressingly routine.

We saw people of privilege in our clinic, too, people with expensive educations and successful careers who were sucked into that same dark world. They lost houses, their health suffered, and they disappeared from their former lives. Often it took repeated failures at rehab before they recovered, if they recovered.

One of our patients, a postdoc at Cal, fell into this drug-soaked world. Before that, he'd been passionate about his research and happily spent long hours in the lab. But in the grip of this drug, he took a leave of absence from the university and sank out of sight.

A year later, he came back to our clinic, sober and restored to his former life. I asked him how he'd done it. "I had something to come back to," he said.

THE DYNAMICS OF ADDICTION

I have always wondered about addiction. Why do people do this to themselves? I knew why I had started to smoke, but what about other people? In our psychiatric training, we relied on the psychoanalytic literature to answer this question. According to these thinkers, addiction of every kind is psychologically based. It's the result of trauma, or identification with alcoholic parents, or the preexisting disposition to be anxious or depressed and the resultant self-medication.

To test this hypothesis, George Vaillant, a Harvard-trained psychiatrist, turned to the Grant Study (Waldinger, 1973). This study had been going on for decades, starting in 1942. The subjects were male Harvard students selected for their mental and physical health. They were interviewed every two years into their eighties. At the beginning of the Grant

Study, their parents were interviewed also, to assess the parent-child relationships and see what sort of childhood they had. Of course, they interviewed the subjects themselves about their childhoods as well.

Over time, those who began to drink compulsively tended to develop a different view of their childhoods, a darker view that seemed to them to explain why they lived in such misery and why they drank so much. Admiring and supportive parents were remembered as harsh and withholding. It's easy to see why the analysts who treated these men believed their childhood suffering had led to their later alcoholism. Vaillant published his findings in 1977, in *Adaptation to Life* (1977) and later, with more focus on alcohol, in *The Natural History of Alcoholism* (1995).

Heredity has a strong influence on the development of alcoholism. In Denmark, where alcoholism is common and where family records go back for centuries, researchers studied adoptees, along with both sets of their parents, biological and adoptive (Goodwin, 1977). They followed the subjects and both sets of parents for decades. Those whose biological parents developed alcoholism at some point were far more likely to become alcoholic themselves than those whose biological parents did not. It made no difference whether the adoptees had contact with their biological parents or not. And it made no difference whether the adoptive parents ever drank alcoholically. It seemed that the risk of becoming alcoholic is more a matter of nature and less of nurture.

I have always wondered how this worked. What can you inherit that would increase your risk? Listening to the people in our alcohol support groups, I realized how many had a high tolerance for alcohol. I heard things like "I could drink everyone under the table." A number of people told us the first time they tasted alcohol, they drank until they passed out, and when they woke up the next day, they couldn't wait to repeat the experience. Perhaps, I thought, you can inherit the ability to drink large quantities of alcohol while still enjoying the feeling and still be functioning.

Human beings have been living with alcohol for so long that we've developed a special metabolic pathway to deactivate and remove this substance. We have a dedicated set of liver enzymes that rapidly degrade any alcohol we ingest (Thurman, 1977). But some people are born with a malfunction in one of these enzymes. Due to this genetic difference, even a small amount of alcohol leaves them flushed or nauseated. I will always remember a student in one of the many seminars I taught who had this experience: "Ugh," she said, "if I have two drinks, I fall out of my chair." *What a perfect example*, I thought, *of someone who will never become alcoholic.*

Of course, it's not this simple. When I see a new patient whose problem is with alcohol, I always ask when their drinking became a problem. Many begin to drink addictively after a great loss, something that left them isolated and lonely. Often it was the loss of a spouse. Or it's the advent of retirement, which left them suddenly disconnected from a large part of their former community. They would feel unexpectedly sad, even depressed, and drink more. I imagine the fellowship that people experience in the 12-step groups must be part of their healing power.

CANNABIS AND HUMAN HEALTH

To complete the VA fellowship, each of us wrote a scholarly paper on some topic related to substance abuse. Or substance use, in the case of illicit drugs. I wrote about the effects of cannabis on human health. I knew it gave you the "munchies." I knew it slowed your thinking and interfered with memory. And sometimes caused gynecomastia (abnormal breast development) in men. It didn't seem to be very addictive; many people didn't actually enjoy it. I knew THC, the primary intoxicant in marijuana, was fat soluble and therefore crossed the blood-brain barrier easily. If you smoke it, you feel the effect right away. Also, I knew it stays in the brain for days or even weeks, collecting in the white matter and slowly being released. For a heavy user, this means that even after many days since the last use, a drug screen may still come out positive.

Researchers used flight simulators to test the effects of marijuana versus alcohol on individuals flying a plane. The subjects were ten certified pilots. Those intoxicated with alcohol tended to be reckless and have crashes. Those intoxicated with marijuana tended to become distracted. They forgot to look at the fuel gauge and ran out of fuel midair (Janowsky, 1976).

What I was curious about was marijuana's alleged propensity for causing psychosis. At Berkeley we joked about *Reefer Madness* (the title of a 1930s B movie), which we'd never seen despite the fact that most people we knew had used marijuana. Still, I found that serious study had been devoted to this question, and the answer was unequivocal. Cannabis can precipitate a first episode of what later proves to be schizophrenia or other psychotic illness (Ksir, 2016). But so can going to war, or starting college, or breaking up with your girlfriend. But on its own, it can't cause lasting psychosis. The researchers concluded that cases of "reefer madness" were perhaps precipitated by the use of LSD.

That sent me back into the stacks of our capacious library, searching for evidence that LSD can truly cause psychosis. I remembered Pink Cloud, a homeless man living with us at Barrington Hall in Berkeley. Pink Cloud drifted silently through our large house, avoided eye contact, and interacted with us just enough to get fed. People said that Pink Cloud had blown his mind on acid, and no one doubted it.

But like marijuana, LSD was found not to cause permanent psychosis, only to touch off psychotic episodes in people who were already susceptible (Hays and Tilley, 1973). I realized Pink Cloud had not "blown his mind on acid," as we assumed, but was most likely a refugee from the shuttered state hospitals. Whatever the case, he found asylum with us at Barrington Hall.

CHAPTER 6

Treating Psychosis in Private Practice

THE WOMAN WHO THREATENED TO KILL KIDS

After five years I left my Kaiser job, took a year off to care for our new baby, and thought about my next step. After six years of psychiatric training plus one year at Highland Hospital on a locked psychiatric ward and another long stretch seeing crack addicts at Kaiser, Oakland, I imagined that private practice would be a welcome relief from such intense suffering. So I opened a part-time private practice with an office in Walnut Creek, a distant suburb of San Francisco. I had a window that looked out into the branches of a large live oak. The streets were clean. I thought I would stay there for a long time.

I'd been there for a few years when Betty was referred to me by a colleague with a warning that she was "pretty disturbed." I didn't hesitate. I'd never been afraid of my patients.

"No problem," I said. "I'd be happy to see her."

Betty was a slight, dark-haired woman in her early thirties. She dressed casually and wore her hair in a ponytail that reached halfway down her back.

"I'm here because my ex-friend is driving me crazy," she said. "Her name is Linda. Linda McKay."

"I'm sorry to hear that," I said. "How is she driving you crazy?"

"We're in competition. We've always been in competition, even when we were little kids."

That sounded normal to me and quite common, even between best friends. But the competition Betty meant related to having children. Linda had three by now, all under five.

"But she's selfish. She won't let me have any kids," Betty told me, as her dark eyes filled with tears.

Suddenly I remembered what my colleague had told me about Betty. *"She's pretty disturbed."*

"How is Linda doing that?" I asked carefully.

"By having babies, of course."

Betty and Linda had grown up together but drifted apart after Linda left home. When Linda got married and started her family, Betty had her first psychotic break and was hospitalized for a week. She refused follow-up care and managed to keep her job as a file clerk, but her social life deteriorated. She had brief relationships with men and was sexually active but had never gotten pregnant.

As I listened to this story, I felt immensely sad for Betty, although her own expression was one of set determination rather than sadness.

I saw Betty for a month and tried to understand more about who she was. But she seemed uninterested in talking about anything except Linda and how her ex-friend was ruining her life.

One day she said, "I'm going to kill her," looking straight at me with that same determined look. "Her and all her children."

I stared at her, overcome with horror.

When she saw my look, she relaxed and smiled at me. "It's the only time I feel happy," she said. "When I think about that."

I asked if she had a plan for how to do these murders and she said she'd use a gun, of course.

"Do you have a gun?" I asked.

"No, but they're easy to get," she assured me with a relaxed smile that made me even more anxious.

"You're serious about this," I said.

"Oh, yes. Totally serious."

I paused, gathering my thoughts before explaining about the Tarasoff warning. "I have to tell you. Under the law, if we hear a patient tell us they're going to kill someone—a specific person—and they're serious, we have to contact that person and warn them."

She shrugged. "Go ahead."

By that time, I had enough identifying information about Linda— her last name and where she lived—to track down a phone number for her. I called the number, but it had been disconnected, with no new number. I wondered if Linda had moved out of the state or was just lying low. She seemed to have disappeared herself. It made me still more convinced of Betty's seriousness.

In California, we can call a number for an office that regulates gun sales. I called that office, explained about my patient and her threat, and requested that they add her to the "do not sell firearms" list. The man I spoke to checked while I waited. When he came back on the line, he said they already had her on the list. Someone else was worried, too.

I had the feeling the only responsible thing to do was to continue seeing Betty—or maybe I didn't know what else to do. But while I was trying to figure it out, she began a campaign to get me to have lunch with her. I explained that I couldn't do that; it was unethical. She brushed that aside.

The next time we met, she said, "I'm going to force you to have lunch with me." I knew she couldn't do that, but it was weird and it made me uneasy.

Then she told me about a dream she'd had the night before. It was about her and Linda. The two of them were talking, sitting opposite one another. As they talked, she picked up her purse and threw it at Linda. Then in the dream Linda became me.

She must have seen my look of fear as she smiled serenely, reached for her purse, and heaved it across the room at me.

It freaked me out. All the warning signs I'd been staving off were flashing red, and I finally saw them. Betty was merging Linda with me, and she had turned her psychotic focus on me now. I knew that Linda was gone—I'd tried to reach her to give her the Tarasoff warning. But I was right here, ready and available.

"I can't see you anymore," I told Betty. "You're talking about murder. You're scaring me."

That was the last time I saw Betty in my office, but I was afraid of her for a long time. Every day as I sat in my office in Walnut Creek, I wondered if she was on the other side of the door.

What frightened me the most was that I had two young children of my own. I lived in a different city, but we are easy to find. I found myself mentioned on the internet a number of times, including several with my home address. My daughters could walk out of our house and be shot.

Although I never saw Betty again, I worried about her for years. And I learned something about how to work with people who suffered from psychotic illness: sometimes it's safer to spread around the helper identity, to be part of a clinic or a hospital staff. You have people around you with whom to share your impressions and who can help you make judgments. And you're not a lonely target, easy to zero in on, as I was with Betty in Walnut Creek.

TEN THOUSAND HOURS OF LISTENING

When I was in training as a new psychiatry resident, learning how to do psychotherapy and looking for teachers to help me with my cases, I had many possible candidates to choose from. I chose the most easygoing, least judgmental, and all-around fun-to-be-with teachers. Some were analysts (psychoanalysts) and others were not. I discovered that although the analysts weren't always the most fun, they uniformly understood my cases better than the others did and had the most useful advice. They heard the hours I presented with special insight and could point out whether I was stuck and why or if I was about to lose the patient and give me the advice I needed to rescue the situation.

After a while I found my own therapist—an analyst, of course. Then I began taking the yearlong trainings sponsored by the San Francisco Psychoanalytic Institute to learn for myself how to listen more effectively.

Right away I realized I was out of the loop. Each week, as we listened to each other's therapy hours, there were moments when the whole group—except for me—would burst into laughter. I was always mystified, wondering what I'd missed. Nobody had said anything funny. Later, as I persisted in these courses, I too joined in the laughter.

I realized these moments of hilarity concerned what was unspoken between the patient and the therapist. We might hear an earnest effort by the kindly patient not to hurt the therapist's feelings, and the therapist's earnest effort to forge ahead, completely unaware that the patient was trying to voice a complaint. We laughed because we had all been there—we'd been that clueless therapist, earnestly forging ahead.

The act of confiding to another or being a confidant creates a strong bond. We become attached to our patients and they to us. We care very much about how things go in our work together. A large part of learning how to listen is learning how to hear what we don't want to hear. For example, we don't want to hear that the patient is unhappy with us and wants to leave. Or that the patient is angry with us. Or that we're not helping the patient.

So the other part of psychoanalytic listening is listening to ourselves. For instance, being aware of what we're afraid of, what offends us, or what we're wishing. We have to discern which it is. And we have to tolerate uncertainty.

It takes years to become a psychoanalyst. Although we've already spent years learning how to be therapists, we go back to school and spend five or six more years learning how to be analysts. We're learning the art of psychoanalytic listening, and it takes about 10,000 hours of practice, counting the years in professional training prior to starting analytic training.

To become a psychoanalyst, you must carry several psychoanalytic cases, each one for years. If you're seeing three people in analysis, four times a week each, that's 12 hours a week, in addition to your regular practice.

When we talk about "hours" in this context, we mean the time spent with the patient, usually 50 minutes. However, as a trainee in psychotherapy or psychoanalysis, you spend at least 10 minutes more after the hour (and more time later that day) writing "process notes," in which you try to record the whole 50-minute session, complete with your own reactions and all the nonverbal communication during that session. In the process of writing those notes, we "listen" again to the hour, and often we notice things that went right by us at the time.

We use these process notes to present our work in our weekly meetings with the training analyst hearing that particular case. Each analytic case requires a separate consultant ("supervisor" in this context), which means three or more hours spent with supervisors. Also we have ongoing weekly seminars and case conferences in which we listen to other people's cases—a few more hours of listening practice each week.

Malcolm Gladwell (2008) wrote that 10,000 hours is the amount of practice required to master a complex skill, such as playing the violin. Counting 40 hours a week, 50 weeks per year, for five years, 10,000 is the approximate number of hours spent by a candidate in training to become a psychoanalyst. This includes listening to cases presented by others, time spent in supervision of one's own cases, and, of course, the rest of the weekly hours spent in private practice. And it leaves aside all the hours of listening required to become a competent therapist before starting analytic training.

Freud advised the analyst to "turn his own unconscious like a receptive organ towards the transmitting unconscious of the patient" (Freud, 1912). He was describing our free-floating attention that (ideally) hovers above our conscious conversation with our patient. This is not always easy to sustain.

When I was a brand-new psychiatry resident, Richard Poe, the lead psychiatrist on the 2N unit told me, "If you find yourself feeling angry and you can't understand why, there's a good chance the person you're with is feeling angry." I think what he was talking about was simple unconscious mirroring. What's being picked up by the listener is the body language, the prosody of speech, and all the other nonverbal aspects of communication. It's the music, not the words. In psychoanalytic language, this could be called projective identification—the way that states of mind seem to be contagious, to osmose from one person to another without our awareness.

When the speaker is stressed and conflicted or angry and trying not to show it, and we've had that experience ourselves, we feel their experience in our own bodies. Often we feel the other person's experience before our conscious minds realize what we're feeling.

Bion considered what gets in the way of listening. He urged us to "enter each hour without memory or desire" (Bion, 1967). He accurately perceived that our sensitive attunement can be derailed by desire and memory. "Desire" could imply illicit wishes, but usually we desire more mundane things, such as our wish to heal the patient, a wish to follow a particular thread that interests us, or a wish to make a brilliant interpretation. Sometimes our wish is simply to understand the patient.

Memory, Bion's second roadblock to listening, is of course part of any conversation. But for analytic listening, the useful memory is one that bubbles up into the analyst's (or sometimes the patient's) consciousness without prior planning. It is the opposite of the predetermined agenda. We want our patient to ramble, and as we follow along, neither one of us knows exactly where we're going. Then we experience the joy of discovery of some insight that neither of us could have reached through a planned discussion.

At some point, of course, we have to say something about what we're hearing. That, too, is a skill that needs to be developed. The watchword is "tact and timing." All of this refers to psychodynamic psychotherapy. Today there are numerous forms of individual psychotherapy, some better known than others. One of the more prominent and well-studied is cognitive behavioral therapy (CBT). Motivational interviewing is often mentioned as well, especially in the treatment of addiction.

No matter the therapist's approach, healing requires an equal amount of work on the part of the patient. It requires a therapeutic alliance between patient and therapist; that is, an agreement to work together on the problem brought by the patient. Even in the rest of medicine, in which the patient presents symptoms, the doctor makes a diagnosis and recommends a treatment, we still need a therapeutic alliance. We need the patient's trust, and the patient needs to know that we'll be available if questions come up. A prescription can be just the beginning.

In analytic circles, we often look for "analyzable" patients—those who have access to their internal experience and can verbalize it. And we look for motivated patients—people who come with a complaint, readily form a therapeutic alliance with us, and work with us in the project of healing.

But what about those who don't fit this model? Many years after I finished analytic training, I began working at a local clinic devoted to people with severe mental illness. Often they suffered from psychotic symptoms—hallucinations, paranoid delusions, garbled communication, and little insight into their inner lives. Traditionally these patients are not considered suitable for analytic work. Nevertheless, these psychotic patients benefitted from having a reliable listener.

Others in the clinic had noticed the same thing. One of our most experienced caseworkers, Deborah, described her practice of listening, on a routine basis, to her clients. She wasn't listening for data, such as need for housing or the level of disability. She was just listening with attention and empathy. When another case manager, much newer to the profession, asked anxiously if that was required, Deborah said it was her practice. "It's part of their medicine," she said.

Another case manager, also with many years of experience but not trained as a psychotherapist, set aside ten minutes every week for a particular client to call her. If he did, she would listen for those ten minutes. "He tells me the same thing every time," she said. "But it seems to help. When I stopped, he got worse."

Psychoanalysis has changed greatly since the days of Freud. Today most analysts are women, not men. Most of us are psychologists, psychiatric social workers, or marriage and family therapists. Very few of us are psychiatrists. We treat Freud in the affectionate but amused way we might treat a great-uncle whose portrait hangs on the wall. A Victorian gentleman who was shocked by the brutality of World War I, and in 1938 fled the Nazis for the friendlier climate of London.

Perhaps the biggest change is in what we think about as we work. Rarely does any of us talk about childhood sexuality, the Oedipus complex, penis envy, or similar staples of "Freudian" thought. We don't find it very useful. For me, the important idea we've retained is our belief in the power of empathic listening.

A Psychodynamic Approach to the Treatment of Psychosis: Chris

Everything blew up for Chris in organic chemistry class. Shaky after another sleepless night, he reached too fast for the sulfuric acid and watched in horror as the glass vial skittered off the workbench and shattered on the floor.

His lab partner leapt back from the spreading pool. "What the fuck, Chris!" The lab instructor was by his side in seconds, shouting directions.

Somebody muttered "loser" loud enough for Chris to hear. The whole class had gathered, peering around the benches at the viscous pool spreading across the floor. As the first whiff of acid fumes filled his nose and stung his eyes, he heard the same voice again, from the back of the room. "Thanks a lot, loser."

His face grew hot, and he knew he'd turned bright red. In a daze, he pulled on the latex gloves and cautiously swept up the mess. As he followed up with a wet mop, somebody else called from the back of the room, "Asshole." He looked around, trying to see who it was, but everyone acted as if they had gone back to work and weren't paying any attention to him.

The cruelty of it made him furious. It never occurred to him that he was hallucinating.

He tried to start over the lab, with a new vial of sulfuric acid, but he couldn't concentrate. The instructor was erasing chemical reactions from the board when Chris approached him.

"I'm done," he said.

The teacher looked around in surprise. "Already?"

"No, I mean done with the class. Not coming back."

Chris hated organic chemistry. It was just for premeds, and he had no desire to be a doctor. That was his father's dream, not his. Unfortunately his father called from home that evening to arrange for pickup at the airport when Chris flew in from Houston. "How're you doing in organic?" he asked.

"I dropped the class today."

At that his father exploded. "All the money we've spent," his father bellowed. "You're 22; you still haven't graduated!" Chris held the phone away from his ear. "You're majoring in loser. How to be a loser in life."

Chris said nothing. It wasn't the first time his father had called him a loser.

This is what I pictured later, as I listened to Chris and read his medical records. He was referred to me by Dr. M., his second psychiatrist since he'd returned home. "He's not clearing," she said, meaning he was still having psychotic symptoms. She had tried to get Chris to take his Zyprexa, the antipsychotic he'd been prescribed in Houston, but he didn't believe in medication.

"I'm referring him to you because I'm focusing my practice on analytic cases," she told me apologetically. "I'll send you his records from the Houston hospital. They thought he was bipolar."

I hung up the phone, feeling a mixture of curiosity and dread. I would be the third psychiatrist in three weeks to see Chris.

I understood Dr. M.'s apologetic tone. I was in the midst of analytic training, and like Dr. M., I wanted to do more psychoanalysis. Also, treating a psychotic patient requires extra work: collaboration with family members and with a wide variety of other professionals. Reading reports, sending for documents, consultation with other clinicians, calling in prescriptions, ordering lab work, and chasing down lab results. None of these are "billable." You do it on your own time, whenever the need arises.

It feels more urgent than with a less-disturbed patient. As Zaheer writes, people with serious mental illness have a high rate of suicide, twenty times the expected rate in the early stages of schizophrenia (Zaheer, 2020). Grotstein writes that schizophrenia is primarily a disorder of meaninglessness: all that we take for granted to make sense of the world is gone (Grotstein, 1990). The experience is like falling into a "black hole," he writes. This inability to sense what's meaningful and what isn't leaves the patient in a terrifying and lonely world, where no one can be trusted. I knew how hard it would be to engage this patient in treatment.

To my surprise, Chris was early for his first appointment with me. When I saw the light go on in my office, I felt hopeful until I went out to meet him and saw that his mother sat across from him in our tiny waiting room. He didn't look happy. I wondered if she had brought him because she didn't trust him to get to my office on his own. He had the look of a prisoner.

Chris was rail thin. He was tall, with a stoop that gave him a hangdog look. He was pale, with freckles and thinning red hair cut short.

In my office he sat silently, staring at my rug. When I asked, he said he was doing fine. After a pause I asked, "What happened that you ended up in the hospital?"

"My roommate took me to the hospital," he told me. "But there's nothing wrong with me. I can take care of myself."

I nodded, wondering why I'd agreed to take him.

"I don't believe in drugs. I keep myself in balance with exercise. I just stopped sleeping."

He paused for a long time while I waited for him to speak. Finally he said, "There was a test. To see what sort of human being I was. I failed."

"You failed?"

"My roommates were talking about me. Saying crude things."

"Crude things like . . ."

"Like, 'Chris is an asshole.'"

"How horrible!" I said.

"I'm selfish, I think I know more than I do, and I'm not open to other people." Then he fell silent again.

The voices he heard sounded like hallucinations to me. His conviction about the test sounded delusional. But he was sharing his experiences with me, and I wasn't going to argue.

When I asked if I could talk with Dr. M. and with the pastor who'd seen him in Houston, he readily agreed and signed the information release forms.

I was happily surprised when he returned the next day as we'd planned, this time without his mother. He told me he'd started Depakote, a mood stabilizer he'd been prescribed, "but it's raising my blood pressure. I can feel it."

75

You can't feel your blood pressure going up, but I said nothing. I interpreted it as a metaphor. I thought he was angry about what had happened to him. Understandably. He was stopped in his tracks by this illness, just when he was finding his way forward in life. Terrible, rotten luck. *There's no justice*, I thought.

"It's making me sleepy," he added. "I'm whimsical. It's interfering with my imagination."

I'd never heard it put that way, but it suggested a side of Chris that made me feel hopeful. In the midst of this disaster, he remembered his old self—a creative self, perhaps.

"Everyone at Rice knew who I was. They think I'm girlish."

"I doubt that," I said. If I had let that pass, he might think I agreed.

"They made a test—a prank—a joke prank. I had a freak-out in chemistry."

"A joke?" *What kind of cruel joke would that be?* I wondered.

"They talk about my inadequate performance."

I was starting to get that fuzzy feeling I get when I'm struggling to follow the logic of someone with a thought disorder. It feels like my mind is slipping. As if this disordered thinking is contagious. And in fact, it is.

Bion writes that a person in the grip of psychosis communicates by means of projective identification (1962). That is, the anguished person's unbearable emotional state manifests in the listener, as if by osmosis. As I listened to Chris struggling to make sense of his experience and as I tried and failed to follow his logic, I joined him in experiencing an inability to think.

Rosenfeld agrees that projective identification can be a means of communication and that the analyst can use the patient's projection "to feel and understand his experiences and to contain them" (Rosenfeld, 1987). This was my job: to tolerate that frightening state of mind and to sit with it.

It's not easy. Describing himself with wonderful humility as "the eagerly hopeful analyst," Searles writes of "the full agony of my subjective incompetence, impotence, and malevolence which the work with these patients evokes in me" (Searles, 1976).

To clear my mind, I spent the next hour reading Chris's records. The psychiatrist who'd seen him in the Houston hospital ER wrote that Chris was in restraints during his examination. He had assaulted two nurses, the doctor wrote. Security was called, and he was wrestled into restraints. I tried to imagine Chris assaulting anyone and concluded he'd probably pushed the nurses as they tried to get him to take medication. That could count as assault.

The examining psychiatrist wrote, "Patient showed extreme anxiety, psychosis with auditory hallucinations," and admitted him to the psychiatric ward. Chris became irate and demanded a lawyer to get him out. "There's nothing wrong with me," he said. He just needed exercise and sleep. He was a long-distance runner, and he ran many miles every day around the large Rice University campus.

In the hospital, he refused all medications except for a sedative at bedtime and one dose of Haldol in exchange for the removal of the restraints. He was held for five days in that hospital before he was discharged. As soon as he was free, he flew back home.

When I reached her on the phone, Dr. M. said, "It came on so suddenly, we thought it was drug toxicity. But all the drug screens were negative."

"The hospital note said he was 'grandiose,'" I told her. "What did they see as grandiose?"

"He kept insisting everyone knew him at Rice."

We were all struggling with the usual problem of diagnosis and the wish to find that Chris had an easily treatable illness. Grandiosity often goes along with bipolar disorder, which has a better prognosis than schizophrenia. Uncomplicated drug toxicity would have the best outlook.

I reached the Methodist pastor in Houston, grateful for his availability. Ministers often have training in mental health counseling to prepare them for their pastoral care duties, and this pastor seemed especially well-versed.

"Chris was emotionally volatile, hypomanic at times, possibly delusional, with no vocabulary to express his feelings," the pastor said. All along Chris had been isolated and unhappy, depressed even at his best. "At the end he felt broken and unfixable."

His last words conveyed so much pain and hopelessness that finally I couldn't walk away. For better or worse, I was all in on Chris.

Two days later, instead of Chris, it was his mother who showed up. I noticed again how much the tall, angular woman with her faded red hair tied back in a thin ponytail resembled her son. She clutched a file folder in her hand. Her serious look told me to skip the pleasantries and get right to the point.

"I brought you a family tree," she began, opening the folder and handing me a diagram showing Chris's many relatives with psychotic disorders—schizophrenia, schizoaffective disorder, and bipolar disorder with episodes of psychosis. Clearly she understood that schizophrenia has some genetic components (Kendler and Diehl, 1993). She watched me closely as I studied the family tree. I imagined the dread she must be feeling.

If Chris had not been psychotic—if he'd been in touch with reality and aware of his need for treatment—I would have declined to meet with his mother. Chris was a young man, not a child.

But at that point, he was severely regressed and had no insight into his need for help. His mother was the only motivating force behind his treatment and I wanted to keep her as an ally. Unlike addicts, people with schizophrenia don't "hit bottom" and realize that they need treatment— as Perkins (2005) and Marshall (2011) write, they just continue getting worse. So I met with her that day, grateful for her involvement.

"Chris has been in therapy for years," she told me. "Even in Houston, with his pastor. But he's reluctant to take any of his medications."

Antipsychotic drugs can have a dulling effect, especially in the beginning. All of them have some side effects for some people. It takes steady collaboration, often months, between prescriber and patient to arrive at the right medication in the lowest dose possible.

And schizophrenia appears early in life, just as the young person is striving for independence. People experiencing their first psychotic break face an intolerable dilemma. To need this drug means you have a mental illness and need extraordinary help simply to care for yourself. It's a bitter pill to swallow.

For a mother to watch her child struck down by psychosis is heartbreaking. Mothers are prone to feeling guilt about whatever misfortunes their children endure. Whether it makes sense or not, they engage in painful soul-searching to discern how they might have caused their children's misfortune. This unavoidable self-blame adds to the grief and terror they endure as they watch their children struggle with a psychotic illness.

In my experience, it is the mother as much as the sick child who needs support. She, too, needs an adequate "holding environment," the kind of reassuring calm that a mother provides for her infant (Winnicott, 1965). So when my young patient is acutely ill and unable to see the need for treatment, I meet with the mother, not only to forge a therapeutic alliance but to provide support for her. I think this helps her to tolerate her stricken child's distress, providing a calm, reassuring presence.

In cases of severe mental illness such as schizophrenia and bipolar disorder I don't look to the mother as the cause of her child's illness because of my strong belief that these illnesses, like asthma, cystic fibrosis, epilepsy, Parkinson's disease, ALS, and many others, are genetically caused. But this view is not universal.

Freud struggled early on with the question of whether schizophrenia (known then as dementia praecox) was biologically based or, like hysteria, purely psychological (Freud 1894). He divided neuroses into "actual neuroses," the neurologically based disorders, and "psychoneuroses," the purely psychological disorders. For the next two years, he continued to ponder this question, finally concluding that the actual neuroses were indeed neurologically based (Freud, 1895, 1896a, 1896b).

Psychoanalytic thinkers have continued to wrestle with this question. Often they believe that the mothers are responsible for their children's illnesses. It was Frieda Fromm-Reichmann, that usually wise and compassionate analyst, who called the mothers of these very sick patients "schizophrenogenic mothers." "Refrigerator mothers" was also a term in vogue in the 1950s and early 1960s. Most recently Gundersen has cautioned that neuropsychological explanation cannot replace psychoanalytic theory (Gundersen, 2022).

Grotstein took up this same question, attempting to reconcile two schools of psychoanalytic thinking on the origins of schizophrenia

(Grotstein, 1977). Later he wrote that schizophrenia was a "disorder of self-regulation" with a neurobiological contribution (Grotstein, 1989). He mentioned genetic twin studies, abnormal EEGs, and an excess of dopamine in certain areas of the brain, among other abnormal findings.

Nevertheless, without evidence, he pointed toward faulty mothering as the crucial factor in determining the eventual development of severe illness, a view widely held among prominent psychoanalytic thinkers, who cited "a defective holding environment" (Winnicott, 1965), "a defective maternal containment" (Bion, 1962), "a defective background of safety" (Sandler 1960), "a defective background presence of primary identification" (Grotstein, 1980), and "a defective matrix" (Ogden, 1986). Boyer wrote of "maternal overstimulation and ego defects" (Boyer, 1956).

I can see how these convictions would make it difficult for a therapist to feel empathic toward the patient's mother and provide her with support.

Two weeks after I'd met with his mother, Chris told me he was hearing voices every night: people making rude remarks about him. "It was a joke/test," he said. "Everybody knows me at Rice." I didn't think this was grandiose—it sounded more like the nightmare where you've forgotten to wear clothes and you're caught naked in front of a crowd.

On his fourth visit, however, he seemed more alert, more coherent, and more cheerful. The voices, which he'd been hearing since that day in the chemistry lab, were arguing about him now. One would say, "He's a jerk, an asshole." Then another voice defended him. "No, he's okay; he's being nice."

I have always thought that these kinds of hallucinations are based on one's own thoughts—usually the most harsh and hopeless—refracted through a malfunctioning brain connection and heard aloud. The fact that a new voice had emerged to defend Chris seemed hopeful. It matched his lighter mood.

He looked at me quickly and then stared fixedly at the small Chinese cabinet in my office, painted with cranes in flight against a setting sun. "I can't decide if this whole thing—the voices—has been hallucinations."

I wanted to leap up and cheer, shouting, "Yes!" but I restrained myself. "I think you're right," I said, as neutrally as possible. He needed his own space to think, and at that point he was actively thinking.

"The Zyprexa does help with the voices."

"I'm so glad," I said.

"So I've been off the Zyprexa for 36 hours, and off the Depakote for a day."

That stopped me cold.

Later I wondered if going off his medication made him feel better at first, and when he didn't relapse right away, he must have felt relieved, seeing it as a sign that he wasn't sick after all. But he stayed off all his medication for the next few days, and when I saw him again, he was confused and tense.

I thought he needed to experiment with stopping all the medication to see what would happen but on his own, not under my watchful supervision. As neutrally as I could, I suggested he try going back on the medication, and to my relief he agreed.

But he was agitated. "I think my mom is too much in my business," he said. "I need to feel more independent." He seemed annoyed in a way he hadn't before—annoyed with me. I was too much in his business, too. I knew he was stuck in a terrible position: needing such intensive help from his mother and then from his motherly doctor, just when he needed to be self-sufficient.

We'd been meeting twice a week but he set the next appointment for a week later. I didn't argue.

When he came back the next week, he was back on both medications and getting more sleep but "still not feeling ideal." The voices continued.

"I think I hear them when I'm anxious about what other people think," he said.

I nodded. "That makes a lot of sense."

His clarity and insight gave me hope. He did seem more coherent. Then he startled me by announcing that he had a part-time job, starting the next day. His mother had found it for him. He'd be in an office, filing documents. I felt still more hopeful.

At their request, I met with both of his parents, hoping to get his father's support for the treatment in addition to his mother's.

It was a mistake. Chris arrived for his next appointment with me a half hour late, looking disheveled. I realized I'd blown it, wreaked havoc with our therapeutic alliance by meeting with his parents, especially his father.

"I don't need these medications," he said. "I stopped taking them yesterday. There's nothing wrong with me."

He said he was hearing voices when he was in crowded social situations. His new plan was to envision those situations ahead of time and plan for them.

"I like that idea," I said cautiously. "That seems very proactive."

He complained that he was still sleepy during the day.

I decided to ignore his declaration of no meds and act as if we were pressing on, trying to get it right. "Let's stop the morning Depakote," I said, "so you won't be so sleepy." I took a prescription blank, wrote out the new direction, and gave it to him.

I hoped he'd receive this as neutral, adult-to-adult advice. A recommendation, not an order.

A week later he came back with new insight. We talked about where his voices came from, and he could see that they might be his own thoughts projected into hallucinations. But he wasn't convinced; he was still haunted by the "prank" his friends had played on him at Rice.

I presented Chris to my best consultant, Dr. N., who told me to be straightforward with him about his psychosis. "Don't go along with his denial." He advised me to tell his mother that Chris was still fragile and precarious and to help him have realistic expectations. "He's coping with a psychotic level of anxiety," he added.

I hated hearing this. I realized that I, too, was struggling to accept Chris's severe illness, his probable schizophrenia.

At this point Chris's mother called and left me a message. She was very worried about his diagnosis. Chris had withdrawn from her at home, she said, and she had many questions about how to manage him. Her terror and desperation were palpable, as if just the right actions would magically undo his psychosis.

I saw us as a chain—Chris's terror in the face of his psychosis, his mother's dread as she tried to help him cope, and her turning to me for a magical solution. I was alarmed, too, and turned to Dr. N. for help.

Ogden wrote that it takes two people to realize an unbearable truth (Ogden, 2004). One to know it and remain present while the other grapples with that unthinkable reality. Chris's illness was that unbearable truth.

So I confronted my own denial and told Chris and his mother that I thought it was too risky for him to go back to school in the fall; he was still too unstable, and the chance of another collapse too great. They agreed.

Two weeks later it was Chris who confronted me. "It feels like I have to prove my progress to you for my parents to see it, 'cause they look to you to tell them what I can do."

It was a huge step for Chris to tell me this. It signaled to me that he was sturdier and that my straightforwardness with him had helped him to stand up to me in turn.

"If your parents want to meet with me, I think you should be there with us."

He looked relieved. "Yes. That would be better."

By December Chris had been free of psychotic symptoms for three months. I felt the medication must be right, finally, without the Depakote. He had gained some insight into his illness and was moving toward acceptance.

He told me he'd had a date the night before and had gotten a new job. "I'm thinking of hiking the Pacific Crest Trail," he said.

"Wow! You mean now, in the winter?"

He smiled. "That's not a problem. You start at the south end and hike north, by the time you get to the High Sierra, the snow's gone from the trail." He seemed so relaxed and happy about it, I thought, *why not?*

"That would be a wonderful adventure," I said.

In January his mom called to say he was hiking the PCT and would be away till the end of April.

In April I got a postcard from Chris, with a picture of snow-covered mountains. "I'm here on the PCT," he wrote, "having a wonderful time. I can see snow on the mountains. I probably won't be back home. Thank you for encouraging me to do this!"

But in May, just as he was ending his hike, he relapsed and was hospitalized again. I was shocked by the news and struggled to understand what had gone wrong.

When I saw him again, he seemed to be fighting off collapse. He was back on his original medications, and his plans for the summer were vague. Still, we met every week as we had before, and gradually, over those three summer months, he began to use our sessions in a different way. He was trying to understand his illness and how to cope with it.

"This is different from the first time," he said. "I heard voices all the time then. I was totally freaked out. This is different."

He went back to school, took an advanced calculus course, and did well. He said, "I think I could live at a higher level and be happier." After a pause, he added, "I've been thinking about what got me into the hospital the first time. It was finals, for sure. Organic chemistry—I hated that. I worried I was failing. My dad. . . . A girl I liked. . . . She blew me off."

"And this time?"

"Going back home. I love my parents . . . but it feels like failure."

For the next two years, Chris spent long periods of time away, usually for school. Occasionally we talked on the phone or I called in prescriptions to local pharmacies, but when he was home, we met weekly, as we had before. As time went on, the work felt more and more like ordinary psychodynamic psychotherapy.

Four-and-a-half years after we first met, Chris settled in North Carolina and began grad school at Duke University in Durham. He had continued throughout on the same medications, with no further psychotic episodes. The last time I heard from him he was doing well and would call back as needed. He had a new psychiatrist and a new therapist, though, and I felt our work was done.

Chris had an unusually good outcome for a young person stricken with schizophrenia. Partly this was due to his mother: her alertness to his illness, her determination to get him the right treatment, her unfailing support, and her collaboration with me on his care. Crucially, Chris began intensive treatment right after his first psychotic break. Studies show that the single most important predictor of outcome in schizophrenia is the duration of untreated psychosis: the longer it goes untreated, the worse the prognosis (Perkins, 2005).

In 2008 the National Institute on Mental Health launched a study on early intervention in schizophrenia (NIMH, Marshall, 2011). Their experimental design called for a team of four specialists who collaborated closely on each patient's care. The team provided long-term, intensive psychotherapy, ongoing medication management to determine the most effective and easily tolerated antipsychotic in the lowest dose, family support and collaboration, and vocational rehabilitation to help the patient return to work or school as soon as possible. This early intervention, with an emphasis on collaboration among team members, proved to be far more effective than the standard community treatment. I believe that Chris, his mother, and I provided all the basic elements of this early intervention program.

Schizophrenia is a brain disorder, but the young person stricken with this illness brings to it their unique personality. Chris came with an already heavy burden of depressive tendencies and self-doubt. In his favor, he brought seriousness of purpose, honesty, and courage, which propelled him forward despite daunting challenges.

Psychosis after Trauma: Maureen

Maureen was 25 years old when she took her four-year-old son, Tommy, to a Christmas fair. Crowds of people milled around the long tables, craning their necks, and squeezing between other shoppers to get a look at the homemade crafts for sale. Tommy was standing by her side. And then he wasn't.

Terrified, she pushed through the crowd, calling his name, and pleading frantically for help.

The doors to the venue were closed and monitored by guard so that no one could leave while management conducted a thorough search. But Tommy was nowhere. Maureen's brother was on the local police force, and the city and county police made heroic efforts to find the child, without success. The abductor was never caught.

Within months, Tommy's father moved away and he and Maureen quickly divorced. When she was 28, Maureen remarried, had two more sons in quick succession, and tried to find solace in her new family. Her husband, Todd, was an airplane mechanic for a major airline. He was unflappable in the face of chaos, a comfort to Maureen and the family for what lay ahead.

Ten years after Tommy had vanished, a hiker found his remains next to a little-used trail in the nearby hills. Soon after that, Maureen was hospitalized for the first time with a full-blown psychosis.

The doctors thought she was suffering from schizophrenia. She heard Tommy crying and believed she'd been sent a tape recording by the kidnappers, with a ransom note soon to follow. She was confused and enraged, "obsessed with recovering her son," according to the hospital admission history. During the next 10 years, she was hospitalized repeatedly, sometimes for months at a time. Her parents, who lived nearby, stepped in to help care for the children.

The hospital psychiatrists treated her with a series of antipsychotic medications and mood stabilizers with no lasting success.

Finally, she was admitted to Langley Porter Institute (LPI), the psychiatric hospital at the University of California, San Francisco. The LPI doctors diagnosed her with bipolar disorder, stopped all her antipsychotic drugs, and discharged her on lithium carbonate, a standard mood stabilizer. They referred her to me for outpatient follow-up. Despite her serious illness, I would be the first psychiatrist to meet with her on a regular basis outside the hospital.

The LPI doctors also sent me a brief treatment summary, beginning with Tommy's kidnapping. Eventually Maureen herself told me about that tragedy and what followed, but I was very glad to know about it from the start. Eventually I came to understand her as a mother in a continuous state of shock, terrified of having to rely on her own judgment.

I had seen many patients with bipolar disorder. Sometimes it was precipitated by a traumatic experience. All of them responded well to mood stabilizers and therapy, and I had no worries about how this new patient would do.

I first met Maureen in the waiting room of my Walnut Creek office. She was petite and slender, with round blue eyes and corn silk hair. But she dressed in worn jeans and a baggy sweatshirt, as if she were trying to fade out of sight. She didn't look up when I greeted her but trudged ahead of me as I showed her into my office. I had a circular armchair for my patients, upholstered in a flowery print fabric that could spin in a circle. Maureen could sit in that chair and rotate it so as to sit facing me, sideways, or with her back to me. She sank into the chair and sat unmoving, her head down.

Finally she looked up and gave me a thin smile. "I used to have lots of friends," she said. "Till I got sick. Now I've got two teenagers." She fell silent then and the air felt thick with despair.

A few days later her husband, Todd, called to say that she'd become frightened and confused. "She can't remember anything. Like when she got sick before," he said.

We made an appointment for the next day, but she got lost on the way to my office. Her parents brought her two days later, and I saw them as they entered the building. Maureen stared ahead with unseeing eyes, a look of horror on her face. Her parents sat in with us and spoke for her, as she seemed unable to talk. She couldn't remember that we'd met before.

The next day she returned to the hospital. After three more weeks on the acute ward at LPI, she was discharged on imipramine, a common antidepressant at that time. But by the end of two months, she had stopped bathing and speaking and refused to get out of bed. I thought she needed more imipramine.

Unfortunately, a cautious increase in the imipramine propelled her into a manic episode. Any antidepressant given to treat depression in a patient with bipolar disorder can precipitate a manic episode (a "manic switch"), so we try to proceed cautiously.

Todd called in distress to say she had stopped sleeping altogether and was pulling his hair and yelling at him when he tried to sleep. She was undressing in front of the kids. When I met with her the next day, she was hallucinating, talking to invisible people. I added an antipsychotic drug, Trilafon, to her growing list of medications.

It was a year since we'd begun working together, and Maureen was now on five different medications: lithium for mood stabilization, imipramine for depression, Klonopin for sleep, and now Trilafon for psychotic symptoms, along with Cogentin to prevent the muscle spasms common with Trilafon. In med school we'd been warned frequently about polypharmacy. You put your patient on a steadily increasing number of drugs, trying to address each problem, until the drugs become their own problem.

The Trilafon did help her regain contact with reality. But after a week she threw away the bottle, along with the Cogentin. A few days later she became confused, profoundly depressed, and terrified that Todd was deserting her.

"I think I'm so afraid of being left 'cause when I was four I got lost in the grocery store," she said. I thought of Tommy, the other four-year-old who'd gotten lost in a store, but I kept that thought to myself. Maybe she thought it anyway, because suddenly she became silent and seemed far away.

Months passed and she sank into herself more and drew back from the world around her. I thought it was time to try Tegretol again. I knew she'd taken it before and found it helpful. Tegretol (carbamazepine) is an anticonvulsant also used to treat seizure disorders. Oddly, it's been found to help with bipolar disorder as well. The only downside is that occasionally—rarely—it causes aplastic anemia, a catastrophic bone marrow failure sometimes ending in death.

I reminded her of the risk of aplastic anemia; we would have to follow her white cell count with blood draws. And watch for any signs of infection, like a sore throat.

Over the next couple months, her mood improved and I was cautiously optimistic.

Then she was hospitalized once again at Walnut Creek Hospital, this time to have her appendix out. While she was there, she suffered an acute psychotic episode. Although the hospital psychiatrist saw her, I applied for temporary hospital privileges and went to see her myself.

Following my usual routine with hospital patients, I met with Maureen every day. And I got to meet Todd. I think he and I were both reassured to have a face-to-face conversation, finally. He struck me as the sober, solid man I'd always pictured.

That was the last time Maureen was hospitalized. A month later she went to her younger son's school and met with the teacher to discuss his problems in math. Two months later she was going out socially with Todd. She began to think about getting a part-time job, something she had never imagined before.

I wonder if my going to see Maureen the last time she was in the hospital somehow helped her to trust me, to believe that I understood how serious her illness was and that I was paying close attention. After that, she didn't need to be in the hospital to receive reliable attention. Or maybe seeing me acting like the other doctors at the hospital helped her to see me as a real doctor with real doctor powers.

Maureen attributed near-magical powers to the medications she took. Although the imipramine caused her to gain weight and gave her a dry mouth, it took another year for me to convince her to try Prozac instead. Prozac, which came out in 1987, was the first of the new-generation antidepressants, with quicker action and fewer side effects than the older antidepressants. But she was afraid of getting sick again. When she finally agreed, she lost the weight she'd gained on the imipramine and her mouth felt normal again.

Three years after we first met, when Maureen had been stable for a while, she told me her younger son had a homework assignment to write about his identity. He told her his identity was as an athlete. He played baseball, and that was how people at school knew him.

"It got me thinking," she said. "Who I am is a sick person. That's how my kids see me, and Todd. And my parents, and my brother."

"Maybe that could change," I suggested.

"Oh, no. That's who I am."

And the next time we met she told me she was worse. "I can't sleep; I'm depressed again." Her older son was moving out, going away to college. "I guess I wasn't meant to have children—I've lost two sons," she added.

I didn't like it, but I didn't try to change her mind. It seemed she needed to be the sick person for now.

And then she went with Todd on a vacation to Tahoe. "And I slept well." She smiled, remembering. "We had a wonderful time."

But that seemed to throw her off again. From the beginning, we had followed her lithium levels with blood draws to make sure she was in the narrow therapeutic range. But over and over she would develop symptoms of lithium toxicity—she would lose her balance and bump into things, her hands would tremble, and she would drop things, sometimes her speech would become slurred. Often her symptoms would vanish without any changes, and her lithium level turned out to be just right.

For my part, I became alarmed each time. I dropped everything to call her back and earnestly urge her to stop the lithium and get a level right away. Now when I look back on it, I remember what Dr. Poe told me when I began my internship: "If you're with someone and you find yourself getting angry for no reason, there's a good chance the other person is angry." It was a novel idea at the time. But now I think it's a way of communicating a feeling too awful to bear. I think Maureen shared some of her ongoing terror with me in this way. It worked because I became alarmed myself and she must have sensed that.

I don't think her free-floating terror had anything to do with the lithium; I think it was always about Tommy.

One day she told me she was going to Nevada to see her cousin. "I'm going on my own," she said. "I don't know if I can handle it."

I thought of those crises we'd just handled together. Reassuring her that she had the strength to do it might leave her feeling unprotected. Still, I wanted to weigh in on the side of reality.

"You're doing really well," I said. "I think you're going to be fine."

Back from Nevada, Maureen sank into my round chair, leaned forward, and kept her eyes on my face. "My family worries about me," she said. "They think I'm going to fall apart if there's any stress."

I liked that it was her family who thought she was fragile; maybe there was room for Maureen to have another opinion. "What do *you* think?" I asked.

She looked worried and sat back, turning her chair away and gazing out the window. I realized I was pushing her.

But Maureen did have more insight. Sometimes she could identify her feelings of fear as just that—feelings. And her insight freed me to think psychologically about her experience.

I realized finally that her illness itself had been traumatic—the long siege of hospital stays, revolving medications, and psychotic disconnect from everyday reality. In a weird way, it was both a trauma and a source of comfort.

We embarked on a journey of halting progress in which she would make an insightful connection and then fall back into illness and fear. When she was stronger, she could look back and see what had been lost, but that left her grieving. One day she expressed sorrow about how she had failed all three of her sons—first Tommy through her inattention then the other two through her illness. It was heartbreaking but it contained a touch of truth. The fact that she could think this and put it into words spoke of how far she'd come.

And I thought she had a core of excellent emotional health. "When we first met, you told me about your former self—you had a good life and lots of friends," I said. "I thought, that's the real Maureen, underneath the illness—who you really are." She seemed to take it in.

But the next time we met, she backed off from that idea. "I feel like I'm getting sick again—so much stress, fighting with the kids over everything and even with my parents—now *they're* getting sick."

Again, she fell into a period of deep sadness, but not the disabling depression of before. She was grieving. Her father was sick, her brother had moved, and she was feeling the symptoms of menopause. "That's so unfair! I'm just getting well, and I'm already old."

Then one day she said, "I've been thinking. I guess I've used my illness to avoid having my own life. But now I want more of my own life."

"So you can do things and not be afraid," I said.

"Yes."

Her family needed her to be more competent, too. Her parents needed help now, and Todd, who had always been a rock to lean on, was having serious health issues. Her younger son continued to have difficulty in his adult life. One day he berated her for being so absent while he was growing up. Maureen was overwhelmed with guilt and sorrow for all the years she'd missed out on.

Perhaps this was the push she needed to let go of her "sick person" identity. She turned her attention outward now, to her family and especially to her younger son. And finally to her own health. At this point, she was smoking two packs of cigarettes a day, and we worked together to help her stop smoking.

She raised specific problems we'd never discussed before. It frightened her to leave the house, she told me. Each errand to care for family members was fraught with terror. Again, we thought together about the ways her illness had protected her in the past.

After that, Maureen worked up her courage and drove the many trips required to care for her husband during his medical crisis and her son, who had lost a string of jobs after leaving home.

Maureen and I worked together for twelve years. During the last four years, we continued to meet but only once every month or two, instead of weekly, as we had before. She continued to feel painfully guilty about how her illness had made her unavailable to her family, especially her two remaining sons. But it was she who was caring for Todd now. She was his anchor. More and more, she took an active role during these stressful situations as a matter of course, to the relief of her family.

Then she told me that she and Todd had bought a second house in Grass Valley. A retirement house, she said. When they moved, she would need a new set of doctors closer to home.

Maureen was still taking medication—lithium carbonate and Prozac—and I was still monitoring her lithium levels as well as her kidney function, which can be harmed by lithium. We had carefully weaned her off the Tegretol, keeping in mind that she would be vulnerable to seizures for a while. I threw myself into guarding against this potential disaster, a final prayer to the gods of wellness.

The last time I heard from Maureen, she and Todd had moved into their Grass Valley home, and Todd was doing well, as were her two sons. She had settled in with a new set of doctors. She sent me a picture of herself standing with Todd in front of their new house, Maureen looking more relaxed than I'd ever seen her.

CHAOS IN A FAILED TREATMENT: JULIAN

Julian was 18 years old and struggling to navigate the tricky waters of adulthood. I met him when he was a freshman at the local university. His father was an optometrist and his mother a social worker. His parents had sent him to private school through 12th grade, and they expected him to graduate from college and go on from there. But he was disappointing them badly.

Two weeks earlier, he had left his home in Oakland, following mysterious patterns and secret signals from people on the street. He heard voices telling him he had a special destiny. So he boarded a BART train and followed the secret signals to San Francisco, where he was hospitalized briefly at Langley Porter, the psychiatric hospital attached to UC San Francisco. The doctors there weren't clear about his diagnosis; they had considered undifferentiated psychosis and Asperger's syndrome. But his psychotic symptoms improved with Risperdal, a common antipsychotic drug, so they were leaning toward schizophrenia or perhaps severe bipolar disorder. They referred him to me for outpatient follow-up.

At our first appointment, he settled comfortably in the chair opposite mine and glanced around the office before turning to me. "In high school, I was a teenage model," he told me. He *was* extraordinarily handsome— tall and athletic looking, with the chiseled features of a Greek god. I told myself his looks had given an extra boost to his confidence and tried to ignore his odd demeanor.

Patients who see me for the first time after being hospitalized on a locked psychiatric ward are usually ill at ease. I expect they're worried that I'll think they're crazy. But Julian was ostentatiously casual. He launched into a lively description of his art studio at school and then his collection of old radio programs that he put online for others to share, gaining a small following. "I keep myself even with weed," he added.

I found him charming, although I worried about the weed. Later I read in the hospital discharge summary that he'd been smoking large quantities of marijuana in the days before he began hearing voices and sensing the mysterious signals that led him across the bay.

"I'm not so sure that weed is the best drug to keep you even," I told him.

During the months that followed, Julian was able to go back to school. "I stopped the weed but now I feel horrible," he said. He did look depressed. "I think all this time I've been self-medicating with weed and opiates. But now I feel like shit."

The opiates were new and alarming information, but he wouldn't hear of getting help for what sounded to me like drug dependence. He did accept an antidepressant, though, and when his mood improved, he stopped the antipsychotic. And then he stopped all his medications. He spent long periods of time alone in Tilden Park, a large semiwild space in the Oakland hills, "practicing to be homeless," as he told his mother. He brought home a dead bird and later a dead fox. His mother found the fox's severed head boiling in a pot of water on her stove.

Julian shrugged as he told me about the incident. "I don't know why she got all freaked out," he said.

He believed the radio was talking to him and that his girlfriend and his mother were spying on him and plotting against him. His mother called to say that he was smoking marijuana, refusing all medication, and "having meltdowns all the time." As he got sicker, he became more provocative and dismissive with me, too, and less coherent. He wasn't getting better; he was getting worse, and I worried.

The advent of psychotic illness in a child is a calamity for the family. Often the parents split up under the strain, leaving one parent to cope alone. For the first year of our work together, Julian's father had stayed aloof from the struggle to help his son. He had left the family some years earlier, when Julian first began to show signs of mental illness. The parents had divorced, and when the divorce was final, he promptly remarried.

But after a year of leaving Julian's care to his mother, he declared that he would take over Julian's supervision. He called me to report that Julian was doing very well.

Then his mother called to tell me that she and Julian's father were reluctant to continue his treatment with me, as it was too expensive and their insurance was slow in reimbursing them. She planned to transfer all his care to the county, where Julian could use Medi-Cal instead of his parents' private insurance. When she asked, I wrote the requested letter supporting his claim of disability.

Like most of my fellow mental health clinicians in private practice, I never take Medi-Cal. Not because it pays us so poorly, but because private practitioners in the mental health field find that it doesn't pay at all. This is true for private insurance as well. Those who try to make the system work discover they've entered a Kafkaesque world where directions are impossible to follow. They spend maddening hours trying to obey the rules and get paid for their work, with scant results. Later I learned how widespread this practice is among insurance carriers, who often stonewall mental health providers until the providers give up and learn not to take insurance (Brookhart, 2023).

Julian's father dealt with the financial situation by ignoring my bills. He was a courtly man, tall and handsome like his son, and stiff with dignity. And I didn't think money was the issue. I could imagine how frustrated he might be, first that his son was so sick, and then because I wasn't making him better.

Although his father had announced that he was taking over Julian's care, Julian still lived with his mother. At this point, mother and son were battling over his medications, accusing each other of stealing them, hiding them, or losing them.

I sensed that his parents had given up hope in the face of Julian's chaotic mind. And the chaos seemed to radiate outward, swallowing his parents and then me. We were all flailing helplessly. I thought of the many times I'd seen very sick patients at Chope Hospital in San Mateo and the calming effect that setting had on my patients and on me. The steady, down-to-earth manner of the staff helped me organize my thoughts. Our patients felt it, too. It helped them feel safe, calm down, and think more coherently. But none of us had that benefit with Julian.

As time went on, Julian became more lost in his delusional life. He told me that his girlfriend was being molested by her father and brothers and that a footprint on her wall was the final proof. She was being used by her family as a prostitute, he said, but she'd broken up with him over his suspicions. "The last time I broke up with a girlfriend I had a psychotic episode," he said with an air of careless indifference. "I'm gathering information from the government by starting rumors and tracking what comes back," he added.

A couple months later, Julian was seen in the emergency room after an episode of confusion, decreased consciousness, loss of memory, and loss of coordination. According to his mother, this was diagnosed as a seizure, but no EEG was done and no medications begun. It was mysterious. In the meantime, he refused all medications in the belief that they had caused this episode. He said he would call me if he wanted to come back and see me. Finally he saw a neurologist, who told him the episode had not been a seizure.

Julian's treatment was falling apart. I would think we had a plan, his parents and I, but the plans never went anywhere. Julian was going to stop seeing me, but then he didn't. They were going to transfer his care to the county, but that didn't happen either. Instead, I continued to see Julian but only infrequently. He became despondent, hopeless about his future, and angry at his parents for not giving him money for medical marijuana.

Finally his father called me. "He's paranoid and belligerent," he told me. "He's staying up all night, angry about everything."

I said I thought he needed to be hospitalized, and his father did take him to the emergency room, where he was seen but sent home. *As usual,* I thought bitterly. *No beds, even for a young man who is desperately ill, even at a point when proper treatment could make all the difference.*

The next day I saw Julian with his father. "Julian claims he doesn't need to sleep," his father said. "He gets wrapped up in his projects."

"I'm mending my sword."

His father turned on him. "It's a bamboo stick."

"Someone's coming in my room and breaking my stuff."

His father shook his head. "He blocked the electrical outlets with paper and hung a sheet from the ceiling to block the lights."

"So I can be free from electricity."

"You're talking to yourself outside the house."

Julian whirled on him. "I'm practicing martial arts outdoors at night because that's daytime in Japan. I'm connecting with the people in Japan!" He was shouting.

With his father out of the room, he unwrapped the sword, a length of bamboo about three feet long. "Someone abused it," he said, "but I was meant to have it." He'd found it three years earlier, lodged in a tree on the university campus, and he knew it belonged to him.

I had never seen both of Julian's parents together. They complained bitterly about each other and seemed unable to join in the sort of united front that Julian needed. But after another month of misery and chaos, they came together to see me with Julian, who seemed unusually agitated.

"Someone's poisoning my goldfish," he began. "I can smell the malathion."

His mother dropped her eyes and his father looked grim.

I explained that we'd been trying antipsychotic medication with no lasting success, and I thought it was time to try a mood stabilizer. I suggested we start with Depakote.

After a few days, Julian seemed much better on the Depakote, and I told myself I should have known he was suffering from bipolar disorder. But then he collapsed again, fighting with his parents over the medication and then refusing it altogether.

Two years after I first met him, I saw Julian for the last time. He told me his girlfriend had broken up with him again. "She got a restraining order against me." He looked devastated.

I didn't ask what led to that, but it worried me.

"My parents took off my bedroom door," he added. He'd barricaded himself in his room and refused to come out through the door, emerging only occasionally through the window onto the roof.

His parents had brought him to this last appointment but did not meet with me. They had never connected with the county mental health services. Perhaps they were as pessimistic as I was about what those services could offer.

What Julian needed was a hospital bed. He needed the safety and intensity of an acute care psychiatric unit where his doctor would meet with him every day, ideally the same doctor who saw him outside the hospital. He needed the nurses and psych techs who would care for him around the clock. He needed a team of professionals who would collaborate with his parents to contain his fear and rage and despair, to help him feel safe, and to begin the long process of healing. Because he was still so young, I thought he would have a good chance with the right help.

Perhaps if his parents and I could have formed such a dedicated and coordinated team, we would have done better. But a child with this level of illness puts an almost unbearable strain on the family. The parents, too, need a safe and containing team to help them understand what's happening to their sick child and to coach them through the monumental challenges they face. With such an intensive treatment Julian might have understood his illness and come through with the insight and tools he needed to live a good life. I wish he had been so lucky.

CHAPTER 7

Everything Stops

IN 2008 OUR BELOVED YOUNGER DAUGHTER, JESSICA, WAS DIAGNOSED with a fatal heart-lung disease. An exceedingly rare condition, it occurs in two out of every million people, striking young women of child-bearing age. Jessica was twenty when she became ill and lived until her twenty-second birthday.

I include this history to explain to readers who might otherwise be puzzled by what I chose to do with my life at that point. A friend who had lost her son advised me to keep doing what I'd been doing before, until it felt normal again. I continued to see my patients, but it never felt normal again. I wasn't the same person. I was a ghost of my former self, a failing imitation. So in 2016 I went back to school.

THE SCHOOL OF SECOND CHANCES

Four afternoons a week I stood with the other students at the edge of the huge Laney College parking lot bounded on the west by East Eighth Street in Oakland. As we waited for a break in the traffic, I'd glance at my fellow students, and as we hurried across to the campus, I always had the same thought: this is the school of second chances.

Many of us were older, like me. Often as I walked around the campus, I heard languages I'd never heard before. Ten percent of the student body was homeless, and we had a food pantry on campus. But Laney had a wonderful journalism program. And all you had to do was register for class and you were in. For a year I wrote for our student newspaper, the award-winning *Laney Tower*. We pulled all-nighters in the newsroom to get the weekly edition done in time to go to press, and then we'd drive home in rush hour traffic—morning rush hour, that is. It was the most fun I'd had in years.

That fall, the editor of the *San Francisco Chronicle* initiated a "blast" of media coverage on homelessness, and we jumped into that blast with enthusiasm. As part of our research, we traveled to the city each day for a week to hear lectures on homelessness—its causes, its consequences, and what needed to change.

As we sat together in the newsroom to plot out our coverage, our young editor listed topics on the blackboard for us to consider. He wrote "history of homelessness" followed by a question mark. He was only 25, and as far as he knew, the homeless, like the poor, had always been with us. He'd never known a time when people weren't living on our streets in vast numbers. But I remembered when things were different, and I grabbed that topic, intent on learning how we'd come to this terrible place. The chapters earlier in this book begin with what we learned during that media blitz.

It was tremendous fun while it lasted, but then it lost the intensity I craved. So I did what I'd never done before. I answered a recruiter's call, a locum tenens outfit in Atlanta that placed psychiatrists in positions that were hard to fill. When he mentioned a job treating psychotic patients in a rough part of Oakland, I hoped it would have the intensity I needed. Something I could throw myself into, erase my mind, and hopefully help others.

Chapter 8

Service Center in Oakland, 2017–2021

Orientation: Sophie

In 2017, I squeezed all my private patients into two long days and took a job at the Dry Valley Service Center in east Oakland (fictitious names are used for the agencies in these stories to preserve confidentiality). The service center was in a poor neighborhood with a reputation for danger. The week before I started, there was a shooting in the parking lot of our building. On my first day, I parked in that lot, but when she heard about this, our clinic director, Lauren, escorted me to an underground lot that was believed to be safer. Our receptionists sat behind bulletproof glass, and we had a sheriff's deputy stationed on the premises.

It never felt dangerous to me, but the people we served were poor. Most of our patients were Black, as were all our receptionists, the sheriff's deputy, and most of our caseworkers. But it was a friendly place, and in the beginning I had high hopes. However, it was not like any clinic I'd ever seen. In fact, as its name implies, it was a service center, one that provides social services for people with severe mental illness. The mental health care we provided often seemed like an afterthought, not a serious attempt to treat our patients' severe mental illness.

Sophie, whose patients I'd be caring for when she left, worked alongside me for my first month at the clinic. She was a nurse practitioner, and before coming to Dry Valley, she had worked in an emergency room. When she started work at our clinic, she was so appalled by the haphazard medical care that she drove to headquarters to meet with one of our directors.

"We could be sued," she told him.

He laughed. "Sophie," he said. "No one's going to sue you."

Sophie spent hours perched on the end of my side table, her legs dangling, bare ankles crossed, telling me about our patients. Sophie wore elegant low-heeled pumps. As she spoke, she would catch up her long, sleek hair and twist it into a loose knot secured with a clasp. She never paused for this operation, and later she'd pull out the clasp and let it all out again. Before the end of the day, she would have it up and down again a few more times. She had pale blond hair that hung to her waist.

"How're you getting along?" she said one day.

"Okay."

"Do you have time to hear about another patient?"

"Sure." I got ready to write.

"Brandon Wood," she said. "His mother always brings him. *Don't* let her come in with him. They have a very enmeshed relationship."

"Okay." I made a note and wondered about that, thinking I would certainly talk with Brandon's mother.

"Am I overwhelming you?"

"Not exactly. But I think before you leave we should move all these charts to my office."

She looked worried.

"Is that a problem? I can do it myself if you don't have time."

Sophie glanced toward my open door and then ducked her head and gathered her hair back into its clip. "These are the shadow files. We're supposed to shred them."

"What do you mean, 'shadow files'?"

"The only record is the EMR. The electronic medical record. Everything's supposed to be online."

"You mean we're not even supposed to keep paper records?"

She shrugged. I knew that Sophie had two large file drawers full of her patients' records. "What's wrong with keeping this?"

"We're supposed to scan it in."

"Scan it into what?"

"Into the fiche. Here, I'll show you." She leaned over my shoulder, closed out my screen, and opened a new window—the fiche. I scrolled through it, trying to understand. Documents of all sorts floated across the blue field like trash blowing in the breeze. There was no order.

I looked up into her face. "Really? You really put stuff in this fiche thing? How do you find anything?"

She smiled. "I'll help you move the files."

Later, when I took over her caseload, she helped me carry the "shadow files" from her office to mine. They filled two large file drawers and overflowed into my cabinets. She also explained the Byzantine and hopeless situation with medical records from outside our clinic. If a patient has been treated anywhere outside our clinic, there *might* be an electronic record of that treatment. It *might* have been scanned into our system and then stored in the "fiche."

"Sophie, why don't you stay?" I said one day. "We could work together—it'd be so fun!" She looked pained.

"I'm going to hate it when you leave. It's going to be so lonely here."

She smiled then and looked off to the back of my office, as if there were something to look at other than the blank wall.

"Why *are* you going, anyway?"

Her smile vanished and she stared into her lap, fiddling with her clasp before facing me again. Her words were deliberate and careful. "My energy isn't welcome here anymore," she said. There was so much regret in her tone that it gave me hope.

"What do you mean?"

She wouldn't explain. It wasn't coming from headquarters. I knew our boss had asked her to stay and only called in for a replacement—me—when she quit for good.

"Seriously? Everybody seems to love you here."

She smiled and ducked her head, turning the clasp in her hands.

I tried a few more times to persuade Sophie to stay and work with me. She always got a wistful look in her eyes. I saw her running through the possibility once more in her mind before putting it away again with regret.

"Why not?" I asked, again. She was good at her work, and she loved it.

She was always vague. "My energy isn't welcome here anymore," she said again. Sophie had spent two years trying to change the way things worked at Dry Valley and run up against an invisible wall.

LOVE AND VERMIN

Chloe, a young case manager, would stop by my office at the end of each day with an update on the patients we shared. She'd stand in the doorway, tall and ramrod straight, and speak with machine-gun delivery. Chloe had a beauty that was hard to disguise, although she seemed to be trying. She dressed in camouflage and combat boots, a watch cap hiding her glossy black hair.

When she paused for a moment, I brought up Morgan. "Out of nowhere he said he's not violent. I have no idea where that came from."

Chloe came in and closed the door behind her. "He did time in prison for assault," she said. I'd forgotten that. I was still new to the clinic and Chloe knew him better than I did. Morgan did do time, ten months in jail after a fight. It was hard to remember that about Morgan. He was a big guy, but he seemed like a gentle giant.

"I was asking him about his voices, if he's still hearing them. He said yes he is, and they're telling him to hang himself."

Chloe took this in with a look of concern.

A week later she pulled me out of team meeting. Morgan lived in a board and care home, as did many of our patients. These are private homes whose owners contract with county agencies to provide room and board for their clients disabled by severe mental illness. Licensed board and care operators are supposed to make sure their residents get their medications, but this is often a difficult task and often ignored.

Morgan's board and care operator had called to say that he was frightening her, making threats and acting weird. So Chloe spoke to him on the phone and got him to come in.

We met with Morgan in my office. He went off his Zyprexa, he said, because it was making him fat. And his roommate stole all the rest of his meds, so he was off those, too. He'd stopped bathing, very unusual for Morgan.

He told us his housemate was practicing witchcraft on him. "I'm going to *light him up*," he said. Morgan was baring his teeth and twisting his lips side to side, looking fierce and quite bizarre. Maybe he was doing some witchcraft of his own.

We got Deputy Ramos to see him and do a 5150 assessment. Ramos knew Morgan. They went way back. He asked Morgan if he was going to hurt anyone and Morgan looked down and mumbled.

Ramos said, "Look at me, Morgan. Look me in the eye. We know each other. Tell me you're not going to do anything stupid." And Morgan looked him in the eye and promised. We asked him to come back the next day, and he promised that, too.

I told Morgan it was fine to stop the Zyprexa. It does make you gain weight. "But see if you can find the other pills and start back on those. And could you bring them in with you, so we can look at them together?"

The next day he was a half hour late, but more himself. No more worries about witchcraft. Chloe talked to him about the state of his hygiene. He said he wasn't showering because he didn't have any other clothes. She said she could get some extra funds one time around and buy him some new clothes.

He'd brought all his medications with him, and we agreed again that he should stop the Zyprexa, but I asked him to stay on the rest.

Chloe bought him a fresh set of clothes, and the next time I saw him, he'd found a new barber, too. As he sat in my office, another client caught sight of him, a woman who knew him from his old volunteer job. She pounced on him and towed him across the hall to the nurse's office to show him off, exclaiming about how sharp he looked.

Morgan had lost that volunteer job the year before and gone into a brokenhearted tailspin. He was fragile, medically as well as psychologically. A couple years earlier, he'd been rescued by the highway patrol, who found him wandering along the freeway, sick and delirious.

Now Chloe investigated and discovered that he hadn't been fired from his volunteer job after all, merely fallen through the cracks on his shift assignments. He was back at work, going with another volunteer to visit mental health facilities and speaking to the patients, he told me.

"To be a role model for them?"

"Now you're catching on," he said.

Good collaboration between clinicians has been shown to correlate with improved patient outcomes (Mundt et al., 2015). Morgan's case is a perfect example. What made all the difference with Morgan was that his case manager, Chloe, was a diligent communicator. She made a point of giving me an update on our mutual clients at the end of each day. I was already worried about Morgan, after his comments about violence and suicide, and I told her about my concerns.

Chloe had established a relationship with his board and care operator, who knew right away that she could call Chloe for help. And when she did, Morgan was already on our radar. Deputy Ramos maintained a low-key but watchful presence in the clinic, and Morgan knew and trusted him, as did we. When Ramos spoke to Morgan, we knew we could rely on his assessment, and Morgan trusted all of us enough to come back the next day with his medications in hand. From there it was easy to talk with him and discontinue the problem drug. After he restarted his other medications, his psychotic state was immediately resolved and he went on to do better than ever.

Another day Chloe took me in the county car to visit a patient living in a board and care home. When we went out together to make house calls, Chloe would give me a plastic seat cover from a large supply in the trunk of the car. She wouldn't let me sit in the car with her till I'd covered the passenger seat.

"Ninety percent of the social worker's job is protecting against vermin," she told me. Bedbugs, head lice, and scabies were a constant worry around our clinic. Board and care homes are often infested with one or another, and then every resident of the house had to be checked and cleared before they could sit in our waiting room or come into our offices.

Patients were "cleared" by the beloved Dr. Jones, a family practice doctor who worked with Good Hope Medical, another nonprofit that shared space with us. Sometimes I'd walk by the treatment room and see him going through a patient's hair, looking for head lice. It takes a long time, but he was always patient. Dr. Jones was our hero.

We'd been trying to find a way for me to see Sammy, who lived in a board and care home infested with bedbugs. Chloe told me I should meet with him outside on the sidewalk, so as not to contaminate the clinic. "He'll be fine with it if you tell him we're concerned he might give us bedbugs."

I couldn't imagine Sammy would be fine with it, that he'd be happy to discuss his mental illness outside, with strangers walking by as we talked, much less that he'd be fine with it if we explained we were afraid he might give us bedbugs. What I wanted to do was drive out to Sammy's house. We could see him outside. And making house calls was one of my favorite parts of this job. I like to see people where they live, for one thing. And then seeing the board and care homes for myself was eye opening.

But it wasn't my choice. Executive decisions like that were made by the case managers. I was very new and didn't want to make waves. So Chloe and I talked to Sammy by phone, her cell phone set between us on the table, and Sammy on the office phone at his board and care home. The board and care operator had to vacate her office for the duration. It felt very strange to be having such a private conversation with a patient I've never met, on the phone with Chloe beside me.

But Chloe was satisfied. She wanted to send a message to the board and care operator.

"Hopefully," she said, "this will give her a nudge to get the house certified bug-free."

We shared our waiting room and our patients with the Good Hope Medical Clinic next door. Aisha, the Good Hope Clinic administrator, would send us spreadsheets with updates on which homes were infested with what vermin, which homes cleared, and which patients were cleared or not yet cleared.

Aisha was a miracle of tact. Tall and elegant, she guarded the waiting room chairs with their fabric cushions, tipping suspicious chairs forward against the wall. When necessary, she ushered patients out onto the side-walk, where they could sit on a bench next to the door.

She even took on the problem patients, like the guy who sat very close to the young men in the waiting room and put his hands all over them. Aisha joked with him as she moved him to a distant chair. "You *know* you can't sit there," she laughed. Coming from her, it sounded like love.

SMOKE AND LONGING: BRANDON

If you'd met Brandon at 16, you would never have guessed that in 10 years he'd be living on the streets. When I first met his mother, a rushed conversation in the waiting room while Brandon saw the nurse, she showed me a picture from his sophomore year in high school: Brandon speeding down the football field, looking over his shoulder to catch a pass. She told me the girls loved him.

Brandon was 28 when I first met him. His current case manager, Chloe, told me that recently he'd been irritable, withdrawn, and shut down. But he sat across from me at my desk and gave me a shy and slightly embarrassed smile. He confessed that he'd blown it again and was about to get kicked out of another board and care home.

"Too much weed," he said.

I laughed. "How much is too much?"

He smiled and seemed to consider. "We only get five dollars a day. Two days out, two days in." The same problem with meth, he added: his allowance would buy five days' worth, which he'd smoke in one day.

I hadn't quite followed all this, but I wasn't going to interrupt him while he told me about his drug use. I thought of the terrible withdrawal that follows a run of methamphetamine.

As if his thoughts ran on the same track, he said, "I was in John George." I knew he'd just been hospitalized there for depression with suicidal intent. "They found a click in my thinking."

Neither of us knew what that meant, and I wondered if he had a thought disorder or if he was just confused from the THC and possibly from cocaine withdrawal.

He spoke of being homeless in the past. "I want to do it again." His face was full of longing.

Before she left, Sophie had warned me that Brandon "failed to bond" with his first two case managers and was on his third now. And I remembered her earlier warning: "He's very enmeshed with his mother." It caught my attention. My coworkers didn't usually use jargon like "enmeshed" or "failing to bond," but Brandon seemed to inspire an unusual interest in his psychology. As soon as he went across the hall to meet with the nurse, I raced out to the waiting room to see if his mom was still there. She was—a slight, meek woman, elegantly dressed but radiating anxiety.

I told her I was relieved to be able to talk with her, that I had hardly any background history about her son. She pulled out her wallet and flipped it open to show me the photo of Brandon on the football field.

"That's a wonderful picture," I said.

"It's from the newspaper. He was a phenom." She looked about to cry. "But I could write out some history for you and send it—"

"Yes, please."

As I made a return appointment with Brandon, I found myself worrying about whether he'd show up for it. I very much wanted him to like me and come back to see me. After he'd left, his case manager told me that Brandon left our meeting elated and signed all the release forms without any resistance. These forms gave the staff permission to start the process of getting him on benefits, such as Medicaid and Social Security disability benefits. When I heard this, I relaxed. We were drawn to him, all of us. He was obliging and charming, but then he drifted away like smoke. I didn't want him to drift away.

His mother's letter came by return mail. It was written on lined foolscap, and later I learned that she was a first grade teacher. His father was a cop.

Brandon had been happy until he was injured at the start of his sophomore year in football practice. He suffered a concussion that lasted several minutes before he came to. The injury didn't keep him off the field, but his personality changed. Most likely he'd suffered a traumatic brain injury (TBI), which can cause mental changes, sometimes severe. Normally easygoing, he became irritable and given to explosive outbursts. Strange cars began to stop in front of the house, and Brandon would go out and be swooped away. He came home late and smelled of marijuana.

"His dad was furious," his mother wrote. "He called him a drug addict." But Brandon just retreated to his room, leaving his parents to turn on each other. "His dad wanted him locked up for drug treatment," she wrote. "I said no way."

Later that same year, Brandon "threw a bomb" in the classroom. It was a cherry bomb, left over from the Fourth of July. He was sent to juvenile hall, but only after a furious debate between his parents. They had good insurance and could certainly have arranged for a different placement, but his father said, "It'll teach him a lesson."

Brandon came out of juvenile hall using heroin and methamphetamine. "He'd been a good student, but he started failing in school," his mother wrote. He found a part-time job but then his boss accused him of stealing and fired him. After that, he fell into a black hole of despair and spoke of suicide. And all along, he treated his grief with drugs: cannabis, heroin, methamphetamine, and alcohol. Over and over he was hospitalized for depression with suicidal plans. Twice he was jailed at Santa Rita. Unable to watch Brandon's downhill slide, his father left the family and moved in with another woman.

In a desperate attempt to get him into treatment, the family arranged for Brandon to be placed on a conservatorship, with his older sister, Peggy, as conservator. The conservator has the authority to confine the conserved person in a locked facility. It was Peggy who placed her little brother at Sierra Sunrise, a locked facility where they hoped he would get help for his drug problem, where the doctors could focus on him and find a medication that worked. Brandon stayed at Sierra for five months. He was 24 when he got out and came to our clinic for the first time, very drunk. When I met him four years later, he was no better.

Brandon's diagnosis was "disorganized schizophrenia," but it seemed all wrong to me. He didn't seem delusional, just confused. Also, antipsychotics never helped him, even in high doses. And he had other reasons to be confused, disorganized, and even psychotic.

Methamphetamine would do that. Marijuana would aggravate the situation. I wanted to know what he was like when he was drug-free, detoxed from street drugs and off medication. Would he still be psychotic? He seemed a bit addled in his thinking, but I couldn't tell if that was just a side effect of all the street drugs and medications. And I wondered about a mood disorder.

I wanted to stop the antipsychotics, which weren't helping him. They cause weight gain, sometimes massive, and diabetes. And they can cause tardive dyskinesia, a movement disorder that's disfiguring and often irreversible. Most often it appears as a chewing motion that is hard to suppress. I worried that Brandon would develop tardive dyskinesia and shuddered at the thought. But I needed to know, first, what he looked like without the antipsychotic. For all I knew, if I stopped this drug, he might get much worse. You could do that safely in a hospital setting, but in our outpatient clinic, where I wouldn't see him again for weeks, it would be irresponsible.

But there was one hope. Sierra Sunrise could tell us all we needed to know. With all the obvious doubts about his diagnosis, his doctor there would certainly have taken him off his medications as part of the assessment. There would be useful nursing notes, notes from therapists who'd seen him, maybe a report of psych testing from a psychologist. Ideally, I would see a discharge summary by his doctor. But when I asked Sophie what we did to get records from Sierra, she said, "We don't get those."

I stared at her. "Why not?"

She made a noncommittal motion with her hand. "We just don't."

I couldn't understand it. So I began a quest to get his records from Sierra. But when I asked around the service center, I got blank looks. A profound lack of interest. I called Sierra Sunrise and left a voicemail message, explaining that I had a signed release from Brandon to get his records from his time there. No call back. I called again, left another message, and got the same result. It was baffling. And frustrating. I had assumed that all of us caring for Brandon—at Sierra Sunrise and at Dry Valley—were on the same page about our purpose here: to help our clients. But treating their disabling illnesses didn't seem to be part of our mission. It was shocking and demoralizing. For the first time I wondered why I was there.

Recently I googled Sierra Sunrise. I learned that it is run by a large corporation, a company that runs similar facilities around the country and relies heavily on virtual visits between doctors and patients.

Sierra Sunrise is not a hospital of any sort. It's a mental health version of a nursing home but locked. I wondered if Sierra had a psychologist to do psych testing or if any psychiatrist had followed Brandon individually to carefully review his diagnosis. Or to give him a trial break from his antipsychotics. But Sierra seemed like more of a holding operation where he was kept confined and given his meds. Of his time at Sierra, Brandon said only that he watched a lot of TV. And slept.

The last time I saw Brandon, he told me it was hard to sit still during the day. He said he wanted more community. "There's nothing in the house," he said, speaking of the board and care home where he lived. "I want to be homeless again."

"Seriously?"

"I've done it before—four times now."

He turned toward the empty white walls of my office, and his face relaxed. "There's a green valley—you can walk all day and not see anybody. I stayed there a while." He smiled gently, seeing that green valley, I imagined, before turning back to me. "I can do it again."

"You make it sound so nice. What did you do for food?"

He waved his hand in a dismissive gesture, but his tone was wistful.

"I want to do it again," he said. "I want to fit in and be happy with myself. I want to be part of where everything is. Where I don't feel so lonely."

A THOUSAND MASKS

I was just about to meet Erik Bjorn but I couldn't remember a thing about him. Sophie had given me a crash course on all my new patients before she left, but we had been trying to cover more than a hundred cases. I pulled the manila folder and read my note:

> 28 y/o man—suicide attempt @ 6, jumped off parents' house—long history of violence—5150'd multiple times—2015 assaulted man w/ crowbar—Santa Rita, charged w/ attempted murder, incompetent to stand trial—Napa 1 year, Sierra Sunrise briefly (residential facility) till Sierra lost funding, E. sent here.

As I walked down the corridor to the waiting room, I wondered what led to the crowbar incident. A year at Napa—how did he get a whole year of treatment in the state hospital? I wondered about all those 5150s, too: Were they for danger to self or danger to others or both? Were they quick ER visits or was he kept the whole three days? And why, when Sierra lost funding and had to cut beds, did they choose to discharge Erik Bjorn? Were all their other patients even worse off? I knew why he was sent to our clinic: we were the only one with a sheriff's deputy stationed on the premises.

I put on my most nonthreatening face and opened the door to the waiting room. It was empty. From behind the bulletproof glass of our reception counter, Tia motioned toward the other door, the one to Good Hope Medical Clinic. Against the far wall of Good Hope's cavernous common room was a computer where Erik Bjorn sat hunched over the screen. He looked like an overgrown teenager, with wispy blond hair and large, pale arms. Closer up, I caught a glimpse of the screen: a boxing ring with huge, impossibly muscular men, all in costume.

As I came into his peripheral vision, the screen went dark. I introduced myself, and without a word he stood and followed me back to my office. I closed the door behind him, and we sat facing each other across the long table that was my desk. His bulk overflowed the white plastic chair and his round arms rested loosely on his knees. He was dressed in an oversized T-shirt, baggy sweatpants, and flip-flops. He watched me with no expression.

"How're you doing?" I began.

"You have my name wrong." His face was strangely blank.

"Okay."

"The people who gave me that name—they stole me from my real parents when I was a small child."

"Goodness." I pictured massive childhood trauma. Perhaps an adoption and a wish to reunite with his birth parents.

He narrowed his eyes and fixed me with a more intense look. His eyes were bright blue, the lashes so light they were nearly invisible. His pale face was blotched with red now.

I took a deep breath and slowly let it out. "So what's your real name?"

"Mil Máscaras." He must have caught my puzzled look. "I'll spell it for you." I pushed my pen and pad across the table to him, and he bent his large frame over the page, writing carefully. Then he slid it back to me and watched while I read. His lettering was small and neat. *Mil Máscaras.* A thousand masks.

His expressionless face, his grim manner, and his wildly improbable story came together for me as a warning. It fit with his history of assault and his long stay at the state hospital, which these days is filled with people incompetent to stand trial. He was delusional and paranoid. I didn't expect to have a rational conversation with him.

"You have my name wrong in your computer. You need to fix it."

"Okay. I can do that." I pivoted to my keyboard and typed in his Spanish name, but I put it in the first narrative box and left his real name as it was.

Then he did what no patient had ever done. He came around behind me, leaned down, and peered over my shoulder at the screen. Of course he saw right away that I'd cheated, and without a word he turned and walked out the door.

He was halfway down the hall before I caught up to him. I darted in front of him to block his path. "Wait! I can fix it."

He stepped around me and continued down the hall, flung the door open, and stalked through the waiting room and onto the sidewalk outside the clinic. I trotted along, trying to keep up. A passing stranger stared as we rushed by. "I'm sorry," I said. "That was disrespectful."

He slowed a bit and gave me a look.

"Let me try again, okay?"

"You lied to me."

"Yes, I did. I'm sorry. Can we try again?"

Erik sat while I put the name change into his electronic medical record. Then I tilted the computer screen toward him so he could read it.

He studied the screen for a moment then sat back and watched me silently.

I took a deep breath. "So. The people who stole you from your real parents—did they treat you okay?"

"Them? Yeah, I guess so."

This didn't sound like child abuse. "That's good. So tell me about yourself. What should I know about you?"

He stared at me and I felt he was debating something. Finally he let out a sigh, reached into the pocket of his sweatpants, and pulled out his phone. He tapped the screen and laid it on the table between us.

It was a photograph, a headshot of Mil Máscaras. He was a *luchador*, a wrestler in the Mexican *lucha libre*. His mask was a hood that covered his whole head. A pair of black feathered wings framed his eyes. Around his mouth was the outline of a raptor's beak. It was open, as if in a shriek that leaves its victim frozen with fear.

Before I could look too long, Erik took the phone and put it back in his pocket. I wanted to know more but his face warned me off. So I nodded as if everything was clear.

I refilled Erik's medications, and we set a follow-up appointment. I wanted to see him again soon, given how disturbed he was and the fact that I didn't know him yet. But he refused. We compromised on three weeks.

Three weeks later, when Erik didn't show up for his appointment, I worried. So I called Erik's board and care home to see how he was doing and if he was still taking his medication. I wanted to make sure the pharmacy delivered it. I'd been told this home was one that provides an extra level of care. *Good to know*, I thought, in light of his severe psychosis and history of assault.

The woman who answered had a smile in her voice. "Sure, how can I help?"

"I'm calling about Erik Bjorn. I wondered how he's doing, and if he's getting his clozapine."

"Clozapine?" she said. "No, we never got it."

"I see. We've got a problem then."

A pause and some muffled voices, then a different woman came on the phone, authority projected in her voice.

"This is Inez. I'm the house manager. Yeah, the clozapine's still being delivered all right. But Erik's tapered himself off it."

I was speechless.

"The first week was really bad," she added. "But the second week wasn't as bad as the first." Her tone was chipper.

I realized I was wrong about this house and its high level of care. Perhaps it was the only one with an opening.

Next day, when I spotted Erik's case manager hurrying through the back hall, I fell into step with her. "I'm worried about Erik. He's stopped his meds, and they're fine with that at the board and care." I looked at her for some reaction.

"That's how they do," she said.

"Nothing we could be doing . . . ?"

She was walking fast and not slowing down for this conversation.

Our patients get no individual psychotherapy, no group therapy, and no family therapy. Medication is the sole treatment we offer. Now I was learning that writing a prescription can be an empty gesture. Back in my office, I wondered what would happen with Erik. He likely would become more delusional than he already was. I kept thinking about the man he'd attacked with a crowbar. And about Erik's long stretch at Napa, waiting to go on trial for attempted murder.

Usually I ate lunch hunched over the computer, slogging through my backload of required documentation. But that day, I needed to talk. We had to do a better job with Erik.

For the first time, I joined Lauren, our clinic director, and Dr. Wilson, the other psychiatrist, in his office next door to mine. Lauren pulled a chair out of the corner for me. She was my boss, a diligent social worker whose door was always open. I was sure she'd understand my alarm about Erik.

But when I mentioned my worry about him, she was unconcerned. "We can't force them to take medication." She rummaged in her paper bag and pulled out a spoon, then a strawberry yogurt.

I was shocked. I thought it was our responsibility to do all we could to get a delusional patient with a history of attempted murder to take his medication. To pause and brainstorm about how to solve the problem. Perhaps moving Erik to a safer house or explaining the situation to the board and care operator, who was supposed to be supervising his medication.

But my lunch companions were serenely unruffled. Dr. Wilson turned the conversation to trout fishing.

CHAPTER 9

Effects of Racism

POLICE VIOLENCE AND MASS INCARCERATION

Two years before I came to Dry Valley, the *Washington Post* conducted a nationwide tally of every fatal shooting at the hands of the police for that year, a total of 994 deaths (*Washington Post*, 2015). A total of 498 of the victims were white, 258 were Black, and 172 were Hispanic. In 2015, the U.S. population was 320 million, 72% white, 12.6% black, and 16% Hispanic (*Washington Post*, n.d.).

We can see that for Black people, the chance of death at the hands of the police was more than twice the rate for white people. Whereas African Americans constitute only 12% of the population, they suffered 26% of these deaths. Whites, who constitute 75% of the population, suffered only 50% of these deaths. Hispanics, who accounted for 16% of these deaths, were killed in the same proportion as their share of the population.

Another risk factor, aside from race, was mental illness. Of the 994 deaths, 258, or 26% of those killed, were mentally ill. The proportion of our population who suffers from severe mental illness is less than 5%. Being Black or being mentally ill appear to be the biggest risk factor for death at the hands of the police.

Closely related to death at the hands of the police are the statistics on incarceration. Although today Black Americans constitute 12% of the population, they make up 38% of those living behind bars and fully 48% of those serving life sentences. The arrest rate for Black Americans is twice that for the general population, and 30% of those on probation are Black. Native Americans, who suffer similar discrimination, are incarcerated at more than twice the rate of the nation as a whole (Prison Policy Initiative, 2023).

In 2017 James Forman Jr. published his Pulitzer Prize–winning book, *Locking Up Our Own: Crime and Punishment in Black America* (Forman, 2017). As a young Black attorney who had clerked in the Supreme Court (for Justice Sandra Day O'Conner), he was a rising star. But one day he was in court, defending his client in a criminal case. He noticed that everyone in the courtroom was Black—not only his client, but the bailiffs, both attorneys, and the judge. And instead of taking the expected path to fame and fortune, he took a low-profile job and visited his clients on death row, hoping to forestall their executions. *Locking Up Our Own* describes what he found.

A few years ago, there was a campaign to "ban the box." This referred to the box on job applications asking, "have you ever been convicted of a felony/been arrested/served time in prison?" and related questions. Employers in California as well as 14 other states are no longer allowed to use this sort of question as a formal part of the job application, but a brief internet search will reveal such history to any prospective employer.

This can mean a lifetime sentence of unemployment. In addition to the poverty resulting from lack of work, it is also the loss of meaningful participation in society. As an adult, being unable to contribute economically to the household is highly stressful for the jobless person and for the rest of the family. Adult men without work are especially apt to be ejected from the household and ultimately to suffer homelessness as a result. Chronically unemployed men have a poor chance of getting married or staying married. As a result of all these factors, they are robbed of the emotional support and sense of belonging that they might otherwise have enjoyed. This was what I came to understand about AJ when I met him at the Dry Valley clinic.

AJ's Story

AJ's case manager, Chloe, punched in his number and laid her phone on the table between us. She'd been trying to lure him into the clinic for services, but AJ was reluctant to come. This day we reached him at his sister's house.

After more phone calls and false starts, AJ made it to the clinic and I met him in person. He was a young Black man, tall, slender, and full of energy. He began talking as soon as we met in the waiting room and hardly paused for breath. His high spirits were contagious, and I found him charming, if a bit wearing, as I tried to follow his train of thought.

By that time, he was living in his car. He had stayed with his father, then briefly with his mother. After that with his sister, and finally with the mother of his child. I pictured the unspoken story behind this cascade of disaster as I listened to him. It seemed he'd exhausted his family's patience, a common calamity for people with severe mental illness.

At one point he told me that he wrenched his back and sustained a permanent injury fighting wildfires in the backcountry. "I was working for Cal Fire," he said. He was on a hillside, cutting brush with a chainsaw, when he injured his back. "And then I did two more years," he added, and for the first time since he'd come into my office, he stopped speaking. In the silence I suddenly conjured a picture of what he hadn't said. AJ was an inmate firefighter.

I'd forgotten that he spent years in prison. During wildfire season, prison inmates compete fiercely for the chance to leave the prison and join the inmate firefighting crews. They labor anonymously, wearing prison orange, and staying far from public view. It's difficult and dangerous work, but they do it with the uncertain hope of shortening their sentences. And maybe, too, the chance to participate in something heroic. But despite their training and service as firefighters, they have no hope of becoming civilian firefighters once they leave prison. With their prison history, they're barred from qualifying as first responders.

In that quiet moment I realized much about AJ. He'd served his sentence, but he would be a felon for life. With so many other applicants who aren't convicted felons, why would any employer choose AJ?

I could see that AJ suffered from a mood disorder made worse by his miserable situation. He had that delightful high-energy flair, charming but just this side of becoming intrusive. Sometimes he couldn't keep still.

With Chloe, he careened off the walls on the way to her office. He got in her space. He got on her nerves.

We never saw him in a full-blown manic episode, with rage and paranoid delusions. But I could imagine him having blowups with his sister and the mother of his child and ending up painfully humiliated. There wasn't much he could contribute to their support; he would always struggle to find legitimate work. The situation must have been stressful for all of them.

Explosive behavior lands you in jail, too, especially if you're a young Black man. AJ had an uphill battle. But it wouldn't be a story he'd wish to share with me. Nor would he want to tell me why he couldn't get work now or why he couldn't stay with his sister or his child's mother. So I let it be.

We talked about his car. It costs money to live in your car. His registration was expired. He had no insurance. He was at risk of getting his car towed and having nowhere to live. So it was a great relief to me when he reported that he'd paid the registration on his car.

But then he parked in a big box parking lot, and when he returned to his car, someone had broken into his trunk—unbelievably—and stolen all his stuff. He couldn't understand how it happened. Neither could I. It didn't make sense, and I wondered how confused he was. He seemed to be wondering the same thing.

After we'd met a couple of times, I was sure AJ suffered from bipolar disorder, and I floated the possibility of medication. I did this carefully, after it was clear he needed some help. He refused and I didn't push it. He kept coming back, though, and I looked forward to seeing him. I liked him, and his buoyant mood was contagious. As we talked about the loss of his possessions in the big box parking lot and he seemed to be wondering about his confusion, I brought up the possibility of medication again. A mood stabilizer, something to slow down his zooming thoughts so he could concentrate.

It's hard to explain to someone why they might do better on a medication that changes their brain function. You're implying there's something wrong with their thinking. Plus, hypomania is a good feeling, a bit like being on amphetamines. Even if it causes problems, people rarely want to sacrifice such an expansive and optimistic state of mind.

Once again AJ rejected my offer, politely but firmly.

HOUSING AND HEALTH INEQUITIES

Another strike against AJ as he sought shelter with his family members was likely his financial situation. Chances are that they were not well-off and could ill afford to support another adult in their households, especially one who had so few prospects for employment.

We know that after emancipation, most of the formerly enslaved people in the United States were not given the promised forty acres and a mule. In fact, most were bound once again to the land they'd worked before the war, entrapped in a new form of bondage, as sharecroppers. Under this system, the impoverished, formerly enslaved worker was often tied to the same land as before, forced to work as a subsistence farmer while owing an ever-increasing debt to the landowner.

Later, in 1933 during the Great Depression, federal programs were devised to promote home ownership. One such program was the Home Owners' Loan Corporation (HOLC), established to help Americans buy homes (Bailey, Feldman, and Bassett, 2021). HOLC created maps of more than 200 American cities to guide home buyers and especially banks as they doled out mortgages. The banks drew red lines around urban areas that they deemed too risky for an HOLC loan, "redlining" areas with large Black populations. These maps excluded the majority of Black residents from home ownership, since those who lived within the redlined areas were ineligible to receive HOLC loans. Instead, they were subject to predatory loan practices that enriched the lenders but impoverished the borrowers. While whites were given a strong hand up, with the significant boost to their own wealth and security, Blacks were denied such assistance. Few ever had the benefit of home ownership. Their neighborhoods fell into disrepair, and they were deprived of the asset most essential to intergenerational wealth transfer: a home to pass on to the next generation.

Redlining, approved by the federal government, validated other discriminatory housing practices such as undervaluing homes in Black neighborhoods and restrictive covenants, which forbade home sales to selected populations deemed unworthy, especially Black buyers. Such legally sanctioned racial discrimination also encouraged mob violence when Black families moved into white neighborhoods.

Although the Fair Housing Act of 1968 officially outlawed redlining, its legacy continues. We see it in the dilapidated state of formerly redlined neighborhoods where poverty and lack of opportunity weigh on these areas. Many live in food deserts and lack such essentials as proper home repair, decent schools and roads, bus service, garbage collection, shade trees and other greenery, and opportunities for employment.

Health disparities between Blacks and whites are common knowledge. Such disparities have been assumed to result from well-known health risks such as poor diet, lack of exercise, smoking, and low socioeconomic status (SES). Public health initiatives have been aimed at improving education and raising the socioeconomic status of African Americans. However, as noted by Simons and his colleagues, these strategies have been helpful for poor whites but not for the Black population (Simons et al., 2018). In some ways, life has been getting worse for African Americans, not better (Geronimus and Thompson, 2004). Advanced education, for example, often leads to increased experiences of discrimination and more race-related stressors (Pearson, 2008).

Geronimus and her colleagues proposed an alternative theory for these health disparities, the "weathering hypothesis," which suggests that for Black Americans, racial discrimination is the driving force behind these health inequities (Geronimus and Thompson, 2004; Geronimus, Hicken, Keene, and Bound, 2006). This theory, very different from the standard public health approach, explains why reducing such health risks fails to improve the overall health of this population.

Simons and his colleagues set out to test the biological weathering hypothesis and published their results in 2018. They measured elevated systemic inflammation in their subjects, as elevated inflammation strongly correlates with chronic illness and early mortality. They found persuasive evidence that such systemic inflammation is linked to the stress of racial discrimination (Simons et al., 2018).

Their subjects—400 Black Americans drawn from several hundred families living in Georgia and in Iowa—were interviewed every two or three years from the age of 10 to 27. In addition to structured interviews measuring subjective experience of racial discrimination, they looked at the degree of segregation in their subjects' neighborhoods, reasoning that segregation per se is experienced as a form of racial discrimination.

To understand better how such biological weathering might occur, they tracked the strength of racial stressors for each subject at successive ages, starting at 10 and ending at 27. They found that predictive adaptive response (PAR) best explained their findings, rather than cumulative stress or recent stress. PAR refers to the early experience of a stressful environment stamped on the psyche in childhood and activated whenever that stress is encountered in the future.

So if a 10-year-old experiences racial slurs and other hostile treatment, that child tends to become wary and tense when exposed to the same stressor in the future. Such early programing amplifies the future adult response to the same stressor. In contrast, when their subjects experienced racial stressors for the first time in adulthood, the effect on their health was much less. It seems that early learning fostered a predictive adaptive response, which amplified the subject's biological response to racial stressors in adulthood.

Simons and his colleagues used chronic systemic inflammation as a measure of biological weathering. Such inflammation is associated with cardiovascular disease, type 2 diabetes, osteoporosis, rheumatoid arthritis, Alzheimer's disease, and most cancers (Franceschi and Campisi, 2014). To measure chronic systemic inflammation, they looked at circulating cytokines, inflammatory blood proteins that work in a balanced system to regulate inflammation.

The researchers used a standardized self-report index to measure the experience of racial discrimination among their subjects. This instrument includes examples such as insults and racial slurs, disrespectful treatment by community members, and mistreatment by fellow employees and the police. In addition to these self-reports, they factored in their level of neighborhood segregation. In the United States, more than half of all metropolitan Blacks live in highly segregated neighborhoods.

Simons and his group considered other possible causes of systemic inflammation, such as social class and traditional health risk factors, tabulating them and measuring their effects in their statistical analysis of the data.

They found that discrimination and segregation were significantly related to adult inflammation at every point of their interview process. Discrimination correlated strongly with segregation. Neither education nor income affected levels of inflammation, implying that SES had no effect on this population. Health risks were not generally predictive of higher inflammation, with the exception of acute illness and high alcohol consumption. Surprisingly, exercise correlated with higher inflammation, and smoking had no effect.

The researchers concluded that the weathering perspective was correct and that race-related stressors had more deleterious effects on this population than traditional health risks or SES.

Chronic systemic inflammation has been linked to illness in the general population, as well, especially to the illnesses of old age. Studies have also linked it to social stressors such as loneliness, low SES, bereavement, and post-traumatic stress disorder.

But Simons and his group concluded that for Black Americans, racial discrimination trumps all other standard health risks, including class, income, and education as the cause of the persistently high levels of illness, disability, and early death (Simons et al., 2018).

Discrimination in health care is another factor that contributes to the high morbidity and mortality rate for African Americans. In the "Giving Voice to Mothers" study, researchers from the World Health Organization described seven dimensions of mistreatment in maternity care that have adverse impacts on quality and safety (Vedam et al., 2019).

"Rates of mistreatment for women of colour were consistently higher even when examining interactions between race and other maternal characteristics," they write. "For example, 27.2% of women of colour with low SES reported any mistreatment versus 18.7% of white women with low SES. Regardless of maternal race, having a partner who was Black also increased reported mistreatment" (Vedam et al. 2019).

To determine the effects of racial discrimination on the treatment of chronic pain, Knoebel and colleagues conducted a review of the literature during the previous 10 years and reported their findings in *Health Equity* (Knoebel, Starck, Miller, 2021). They found that Black patients suffered a higher level of chronic pain, complicated by poverty and a higher rate of health problems in general, as well as discriminatory treatment. This was certainly the case for Lucille, a young woman I saw at the Dry Valley clinic.

Turned Away: Lucille

The last time I saw Lucille was right after Christmas, and she glowed with her good news. For the first time since he was 10 years old, she'd seen her son, now 24. Lucille was 13 when he was born, two years older when her second son was born. Her brother had raised both her children, and after their births she'd been kept away from the family. What mothering Lucille got was at the hands of her grandmother, now losing her mind to dementia.

Lucille lived in a board and care home. She was a Black woman who seemed younger than her 37 years, with a trusting, childlike manner. She told me she liked to watch TV and eat. She was cursed with a chronic psychotic illness, probably schizophrenia, and it took multiple medications to keep her free of her demons. We had met just before Christmas, and we'd gone over her drugs to get her off the worst offenders, the ones that cause truly massive weight gain.

We weigh our patients at each visit to track this problem and to prevent its evil twin, type 2 diabetes. At that appointment before Christmas, Lucille stepped on the scale and watched me slide the weights along the balance, the resulting number a new high. Her face crumpled as she stepped off the scale. Lucille was guileless. She told me that she ate a second dinner at night while she watched TV. It seemed to her that she needed this to relax before going to bed. But as she talked, she decided she could do without it.

When we met again in early January, she told me that she'd been keeping to just the three meals, no more bedtime dinners. Then she stepped on the scale, and we saw that she'd lost 10 pounds. She was ecstatic. Life seemed very good right then.

That was the last time I saw Lucille. I was away for three weeks in February, and when I returned, I heard the news.

Lucille had gotten into an argument with her board and care operator, accused her of being racist, and left the home. After living on the street for some days, she had gone to the closest emergency room, the San Geronimo ER, complaining that she couldn't breathe and was passing out.

The physician's assistant who examined her wrote that she was incontinent and had bipolar disorder and schizophrenia. She gave Lucille a diagnosis of urinary tract infection, a prescription for an antibiotic, and a list of homeless shelters "with a hope that she finds her way to one of them."

The next day Lucille returned to the same ER with the same problem but worse. She had a hard time speaking more than a few words. The record from the ER shows six separate doctors and physician assistants examining her, all noting first her incontinence, which was thought to be chronic. Also they noted her psychiatric diagnoses and complained that she was difficult, a "poor historian." Nobody seemed to wonder if a medical problem accounted for her inability to speak more than a few words. She was seen by several clinicians before anyone noticed her severe shortness of breath. Although her diagnosis was schizophrenia and bipolar disorder, nobody bothered to get a psych consult. They had our number but never called to find out what medications she took.

The mentions of her shortness of breath and fainting seemed an afterthought. However, after two days, she was admitted to the ER, and a CT angiogram was done. The radiologist documented the time and date that he phoned the ER doctor with the results. The angiogram showed "extensive pulmonary embolism" (blood clots throughout her lungs), a collapsed lobe in the right lung, and an enlarged heart. No wonder she was short of breath. When we heard the story, all of us who'd known Lucille said the same thing: if that were you or me or any of us, we'd have been hospitalized on the spot, in the intensive care unit.

Instead, Lucille was sent out with a bus ticket and instructions to make her way to Highland Hospital. Normally the impoverished patients who are "dumped" at Highland get at least the courtesy of a taxi ride to that hospital. Lucille didn't even rate that high.

It was February and she was dressed in only hospital scrubs. She never made it out of the parking lot. Later that day, a passing EMT crew saw her facedown in the bushes and brought her body back to the San Geronimo Hospital ER, where she was pronounced dead.

We held a little memorial at our clinic for the two patients we'd lost that month—Renee and Lucille. I stood and spoke for a bit about Lucille and then about how she had died. But when I said I wanted to pursue it, my colleagues shook their heads. "That would violate her confidentiality," they told me. "Her family has to do it." Her family was probably notified of her death, but certainly not told of how it came about. They would do nothing.

CHAPTER 10

Board and Care Homes

AEROSPACE SHIPS

Mental health advocates are calling for many changes these days, but more hospital beds and more supportive housing top the list. Supportive housing refers to the board and care homes where most of our patients live. These are private homes whose owners contract to provide room and board to clients suffering from mental illness. Some are licensed by the state; others are not. Those with licenses agree to supervise medications for their clients.

Years earlier, as an intern on Ward 2N at Chope Hospital, it was part of my job to find a board and care home for a patient who had nowhere to go after leaving the hospital. Every morning as soon as we finished rounds, the three of us interns sat at the back of the ward, each with a telephone and a list of board and care homes, calling one after another in the hope of finding one with an opening. All of us had voluntary patients who were in no hurry to leave the hospital, and we had to find homes for them before we could discharge them.

But the first time I saw the inside of a board and care home was on a house call to see Violet. I rode out to the home with Chloe, her case manager. She'd told me nothing about Violet, only that she refused to leave the house. It was soon after I'd begun work at Dry Valley, and I was curious to see what these places looked like.

The home was a short drive from the clinic. From the outside, it looked like any other house on the block, a drab one-story ranch house that filled most of the small lot. A concrete walk led to a door on the street side of the house, but Chloe led me up the driveway to an entrance near the back of the house. She rang the bell and the door was opened by a man in slippers, his thin gray hair mussed as if he'd just gotten out of bed.

"We're here to see Violet," Chloe said.

He turned away and we followed him into a dim room that smelled faintly of cigarette smoke and Lysol. The floor was covered in worn linoleum. The walls had a peculiar two-tone look, beige over white, as if they'd been scrubbed until the old paint showed through. Two men and an old woman sat in threadbare armchairs, each against a separate wall. The woman wore fluffy slippers and a turquoise tracksuit that sagged on her thin body. All three glanced up as we came in.

"We're here to see Violet," Chloe said again.

"That way. In the living room." The speaker, a man in sweats and flip-flops, nodded toward the front of the house, and we walked down a long hall, past closed doors on either side to the living room. The air was thick with a foul smell, and I noticed a door to the outside with a screen door but it was shut. Violet had the room to herself and didn't seem to mind the stifling air.

She was a sharp-faced woman with a wild tangle of graying hair, half-covered by a dirty watch cap. Her pants were ripped from the waistband down to the ankle on one side, revealing another pair of pants underneath. She sat in the center of a large white couch and didn't look up as we entered the room.

Chloe introduced me, and we stood before Violet, who remained seated on the couch and seemed indifferent to our presence. She spoke in a loud, monotonous voice, a harangue, half-preaching and half-scolding.

"You go back where you came from; I got a baby here. No, three babies. I got three babies in me."

I couldn't tell if she was addressing us or someone not in the room or simply expressing her thoughts. She gave no sign of recognizing Chloe, who'd been her case manager for the last two years.

Finally Chloe interrupted her monologue. "What happened to your pants, Violet?"

"It's them rays. *You* know."

"What rays?"

"From the aerospace ships." Her tone was knowing, as if she had special insight into things we'd never guess.

I introduced myself and told Violet I would be her new doctor.

She waved me off. "My husband, he's a psychiatrist," she said. "He's in San Francisco." As an afterthought, she added, "My other husband lives here."

After that brief exchange, we went in search of Maria, the board and care operator. She lived on the premises, providing an unusually high level of care to her clients. We found her downstairs in her dark basement office, sitting at a large desk covered with papers. The air was cold and she wore a frayed quilt jacket zipped up to her chin.

"Licensing is running after me," she told us. "I pay them more each year just to keep my license—for what?"

Chloe ignored this. "We came to see Violet."

Maria made an exasperated sound. "I can't keep the door locked at night because Violet *has* to sleep in the living room. Then she opens the door for *anyone*."

"Why can't she sleep in her own room?" I asked.

"Because of the snakes."

"Snakes?"

"The snakes the neighbors are dumping in the yard." She rolled her eyes. "And the worms. She says her room is full of worms."

The dim basement seemed to grow darker.

"She kind of smells," said Chloe.

"Don't I know it. She won't wash her hair." Maria paused. "The worst of it is she doesn't use the toilet properly."

Maria told us she'd taken Violet shopping and swapped out her filthy undergarments for new ones as Violet handed them out under the dressing room door. "I had to kind of trick her," Maria said. "She wanted to keep them."

I wondered how Maria stuck it out there under such appalling circumstances, how she stayed compassionate and devoted to her clients. The visit left me shaken.

I knew that 50 years ago, most people with severe mental illness lived in state hospitals, known then as insane asylums. When they were well enough, they lived with their families. A few lived alone in residential hotels. Today only a lucky few live with their families. A few others live alone in cheap hotel rooms. But the majority live behind bars, on the streets, or in board and care homes. I began to think of these homes as the new asylum.

When we got back to the clinic, I called the psychiatrist who'd been Violet's doctor at John George. The police, he said, had brought Violet to the hospital after a fight with her housemate. "She stole the housemate's clothes and left them smeared with feces."

I couldn't stop thinking about Violet's fight with her housemate. Her actions against her housemate seemed so deliberate. No wonder the other woman was enraged.

It reminded me of a vignette I'd read in med school about Frieda Fromm-Reichmann, the psychiatrist fictionalized as "Fury" and "Dr. Fried" in *I Never Promised You a Rose Garden*. (Greenberg, 1964). As in the novel, Fromm-Reichmann worked in a large mental hospital (Chestnut Lodge). She was a tiny woman but a giant in the field, a psychoanalyst renowned for her compassion and wisdom.

One day she was meeting with a new patient, a woman who fouled her own clothing with fecal matter. Fromm-Reichmann was dressed respectfully, as always, in her work clothes. As they talked, the patient reached out and smeared the doctor's dress with excrement. The same thing happened in the next day's session. So on the third day, Fromm-Reichmann dressed in scrubs. The message was, "Okay, if this is part of our work, I'll wear the right clothes. But don't think you're going to drive me away." The patient got the message and never again repeated that same attack on her doctor.

But that was 80 years ago, back in the 1940s, when the only medication available was chloral hydrate, that was just for sleep. Forty years later, when I first began treating patients who suffered with psychosis, we had more effective medicine. At Chope, at least, we could see our patients in the hospital long enough to make a correct diagnosis and send them home with appropriate treatment and follow-up therapy in our clinic. During those hospital stays, we made lasting connections with our patients and with their families, who could call on us in the future if need be. None of our patients was as regressed as Violet.

Today, two decades into the new millennium, we have even better medication to offer and a more informed approach to therapy. But only for the wealthy and those with extraordinarily good insurance. And even for those, there are institutional barriers to effective treatment.

Today, 80 years after Fromm-Reichmann worked at Chestnut Lodge, we've gone backward. Violet's state of extreme psychosis and regression is not uncommon today. Her condition is seen as fixed: no one wonders if better treatment could help her. She's simply a management problem, with brief trips to the hospital when she becomes violent.

Maria opened my eyes to what a daunting job it is to care for these clients and why so many board and care operators are going out of business. Today their houses are worth far more than when they first opened them up to mentally ill clients. While their operating expenses go up every year, the rent they can charge is meager and fixed by law. I'm amazed and grateful that people like Maria still keep their doors open.

A Lightning Visit with Jamal to See Marvin

Working at Dry Valley could be lonely, but Jamal was one of the case managers who would sit in my office and talk. We struck up a friendship one day when we were setting a follow-up appointment and it landed on December 7.

"Pearl Harbor Day!" I said, wondering if anyone in the room would pick up on that ancient piece of history. Jamal did and after the patient left, we sat in my office and talked European history, which was his major in college. It felt like a little vacation. After that, he would often visit my office to talk. He was tall, with a shaved head, a graying beard, and a deep voice. His manner was so disarming and genuine that the clients clearly trusted him. I did too.

One day he stopped in my open doorway and said, "Do you have a minute? I just need you to take a look at this guy."

I closed the door behind me and followed him out to the parking lot, where he strode across the asphalt to a large SUV. I realized we were going to see the client at his board and care home. It was a break from the clinic, riding with Jamal and talking politics.

Before I knew it, we were at the board and care home, another spick-and-span house in a quiet neighborhood. Everyone there seemed to know Jamal, and he knew them. I thought once again what a dedicated case manager Jamal was, steadily devoted to his clients without fanfare.

We made a fast trip through the house, searching for Marvin, the patient. As we whisked through the rooms, I noticed the same thing that always struck me in these places. Everyone we spoke to knew Marvin, and they knew exactly where he was, too. They directed us with total certainty but also with a tone of profound indifference. As ever, people milled around or sat and stared into space, but there was no eye contact between the residents. No one was playing games, or hanging out together, or interacting with one another in any way. Yet each of these men knew exactly who each other man was and, not only that, but exactly *where* each other man was. It felt like a guarded truce. Despite the spotless surfaces, the term "warehousing" always pops into my head when I go into these board and care homes.

Finally we located our client and found a place to meet where we wouldn't be bothered in the living room. I sat on a couch against one wall and Marvin sat on the other side of the room, as far away as possible. We spoke for two or three minutes about the most mundane things, but Marvin was agitated, shifting in his chair, with a look of agony on his face. He kept looking off to the side, up near the ceiling. I assumed he was hearing voices from up there, most likely saying derogatory things about him. Clearly he found our conversation intolerable and was desperate to escape. It seemed cruel to go on, so I let it go. The whole point of this exercise, I knew, was to check off the psychiatrist visit, which was no doubt long overdue.

When we got back to the clinic, I wondered what I could say in my progress note about Marvin. I wanted to say that it was a three-minute interview terminated because the patient became unbearably anxious, appeared to be actively hallucinating and paranoid, and that the interview was done at his board and care home, because the patient would not come to the clinic.

I found Marvin in the computer system. His electronic medical record (EMR) was sparse and bland, and I realized I was going to write the same uninformative kind of note.

In that clinic, and in many medical settings today, our computerized medical records are used as insurance billing documents. The service designation locked into the electronic record was 25 minutes spent in face-to-face time with the patient in the office. That was for our bill to Medi-Cal. But I saw Marvin for three minutes at his board and care home. That says more than anything he's told me or anything I can record that I observed. He's actively hallucinating and too paranoid to sit with me for longer than three minutes and to come to the clinic.

I asked around the clinic for help with the computer program, Clinician's Gateway, but no one could tell me how to code it any differently. "Just do it the same," they said. But I couldn't write that I saw the patient for three minutes on the same report that claims I saw him for twenty-five minutes. That would be Medi-Cal fraud. Nor could I say in the narrative that I saw him at his board and care home when on the same form I'm stating that I saw him in the office.

In the end, I hedged my bets. I wrote that he was taciturn and anxious and appeared to be experiencing auditory hallucinations.

I've read notes that began, "Patient seen at his cell door." It's so useful. It tells you how little confidentiality there was for that interview and that the patient was in jail. However, that note was written by a doctor working at Santa Rita, which is funded by the county. Although they use the same program as we do, Clinician's Gateway, their notes are purely for patient care. They have no need to shade the truth for the sake of insurance reimbursement.

As a clinician, I should write the truth—what will be useful for anyone else who cares for Marvin and reads this note or for myself, if I stay long enough to see him again. But I was a functionary who operated a billing program. It was my job not to gum up the works.

PSYCHOSIS AND HOMICIDE

The day I came back from vacation, Nia beckoned me to her window at the reception counter. "You need to see Lauren," she told me. "ASAP." Her voice held none of its usual lightness, and it made me uneasy.

I touched my keycard to the locked door that leads into the clinic and heard the soft click as it unlocked. I could have checked my mail, sure to be overflowing after three weeks away. I could have dumped my heavy backpack in my office, but instead I buzzed myself through another door into the back of the clinic, where Lauren had her office. She beckoned me into her office and shut the door.

"Welcome back," she said, then her face turned all business. "Bad news. Renee is dead."

Renee was one of our "difficult" patients, an aging and fragile woman who propped up her bony frame with a heavy cane as she stumped along. Her fluffy white hair was the only soft thing about her.

"Oh, wow," I said. "Poor Renee. How did she die?" I had a bad feeling about this. Renee wasn't my patient; I barely knew her. So how did this involve me?

"Apparently, she died in a confrontation with Abby." Lauren watched me steadily as she spoke.

Abby was my patient, a robust young woman who was always friendly with me. She was tall and sturdy, but I couldn't picture her as violent.

"Abby would never hurt anyone," I said.

Lauren raised an eyebrow. "Yeah? The police aren't so sure."

Lauren had dropped everything to find Abby a lawyer before she was questioned by the police. "But they went behind my back and talked to her alone." She gave an exasperated sigh. "Can you go see her? See if she was competent to waive her right to a lawyer?"

"Of course," I said. "I'll see her this afternoon."

Renee had died three days earlier, and by the time I came back from vacation, the clinic was alive with the story of this violent death at a board and care home. I heard it from the case managers and again from the patients I saw that day.

It was four in the morning, they told me, but the residents of Sweet Dreams were wide awake, alarmed by the sounds of a violent struggle upstairs. In the silence that followed, Colleen, another resident, opened her door and peered into the dimly lit hall. That was when she saw the knife as it came clattering down the empty stairwell. It looked like a kitchen knife.

A few more residents ventured out of their rooms to join Colleen, and together they crept up the stairs to investigate. In Abby's room, they found Renee's lifeless body, her face battered and bleeding. Her cane lay nearby, smeared with blood. No one could find Abby.

Later that day, Abby returned to Sweet Dreams. Police were called, and she was arrested and jailed on suspicion of murder. From the jail, she was transferred to a locked ward at John George, the county psychiatric hospital. Finally she was moved to Forester House, another board and care home. It was said to have an extra-high level of security.

At the end of the day, I drove to Forester to see Abby. It was late afternoon in February, the air chilly, the sun almost down. This was supposed to be a dangerous section of town, but the quiet streets and tidy bungalows gave it a feeling of peace.

Forester House was pale cream stucco with windows facing onto the street and the entrance around to the side. The garden was neatly kept, planted with lavender and sedge along the walkway.

No one answered as I stood outside the door, knocking and ringing the doorbell. But the door was unlocked, so I let myself in. On a little table in the entryway was a sign-in log, which seemed to be the "high security" I'd heard about. I'd imagined somebody official to greet me at the door, but it was Abby herself who called down the stairs, her voice echoing in the stairwell.

"Dr. Feller, they said you'd be coming!" She bounded down the stairs, ducking the low ceiling to see me as she descended. She was a young Samoan woman, tall and broad-shouldered, with abundant hair that framed her face and cascaded down her back in loose curls. Until that day, she'd always possessed a certain glamour. But now her chin was smeared with white goop and more goop was plastered on her forehead. She seemed unaware of how strange she looked.

I asked if we could go somewhere quiet to talk, and she led me through a large room where a few men sat silently with their backs to the wall, each one locked in his invisible fortress. Abby nodded in their direction. "They're playing games over there." At first I thought she meant board games or cards, and I looked more closely to see what they were playing. But there was no evidence of actual games. Perhaps she meant it in a darker way.

When we found a place to sit, Abby asked me about her chin hairs. "I'm using this new cream to get rid of them," she said, indicating the goop on her chin. "Do you think it'll work? I'm trying it up here, too." She pointed to her forehead. "I don't know if that's such a good idea. What do you think?"

I got that familiar fuzzy feeling that comes over me in the presence of acute psychosis as I struggle to follow the speaker's logic. Suddenly, in my confusion, I wondered if this was really Abby. Perhaps it was someone else, someone who only had her chin hairs to worry about, someone who'd be surprised if I mentioned the police.

We were alone, but I dropped my voice. "So did the police come and talk to you?"

She shooed that away with a wave of her hand. "They're done with all that. Do you think I should lose weight? I think I should, maybe ten pounds."

As I drove back to the clinic to document our conversation, I tried to picture this deadly struggle between Abby and Renee. I believed that Abby had fought in self-defense. If she had started the fight, that would mean she had gone into Renee's room, found her cane, hit her over the head with the cane, then dragged Renee's body back into her own room, and in the meantime had gone down to the kitchen to bring the kitchen knife upstairs. I didn't think she had it in her to do any of that. And why would she?

Clearly Abby was still confused and delusional the day I saw her, preoccupied with imaginary chin hairs while her whole future was up in the air. I doubted that she'd been competent to waive her right to an attorney when the police questioned her.

As I drove back through the quiet streets to the clinic, I mostly thought about the grim scene I'd witnessed at Forester. The residents sat side by side, but each was rigidly isolated from the others. Some wandered aimlessly, strictly avoiding eye contact.

I realized these board and care homes can be a setup for disaster: a collection of strangers, hallucinating, plagued with paranoid delusions. The voices they hear sound utterly real, and their words can be vicious. You might hear your worst enemy in the room next to yours, blabbing your most painful secrets, and then mocking your shame and misery. Or threatening to murder you.

Abby and Renee had quarreled often before their last, fatal encounter. Perhaps Renee heard Abby's voice from behind her bedroom wall, saying unforgivable things about her, as the real Abby lay sleeping in her bed. Perhaps Renee finally snapped and went after Abby with a knife.

The residents of board and care homes are never locked in; they're free to come and go. But aside from a walk to the corner store to spend their measly five dollars a day or to see their social workers and other caring professionals, they have nowhere to go. They're treated like helpless children with nothing to offer. Naturally, the residents don't look to each other for anything good.

Ironically, the story of Renee's alleged murder gave our patients something of value to offer one another: gossip.

When I walked into the waiting room that day, the patients were talking to each other with a sense of excitement. The Hearing Voices Group was unusually well attended that week. The air pulsed with life.

TATTOOS AND TEASPOONS: GRACIE

Whenever I make a pot of soup these days, I grab a handful of clean teaspoons and remember Gracie.

Gracie was lucky. Jamal was her case manager, and he saw in her a lively, capable woman, someone more able than disabled. He found a room for her in a large house with real roommates, not a board and care home. It was with five young men and in a tough neighborhood, but Jamal told me they were protective of her and looked after her. Gracie's new housemates were all young enough to be her grandsons. They treated her like their grandma, and like a good grandma, she cooked for them. It was a happy situation. For a while.

When Jamal first introduced her to me, they'd come from the farmers market. Tiny Gracie followed by tall Jamal, who trailed a wire cart loaded with produce.

Though fragile and delicate, Gracie was fierce with body art. "It keeps the men away," she confided to me. I couldn't tell if she was joking or serious. Her gray hair was shaved off one side of her head and the other half hung down in a ragged fringe.

She told me she never took the Seroquel that her last doctor had prescribed, and it was piling up by the bottleful at home. "It makes me sleep for sixteen hours," she said.

"We certainly don't want that," I said. Like many of our patients, she carried a diagnosis of schizoaffective disorder. It indicates a general mixture of bipolar disorder (mood swings with severe bouts of depression and mania) and psychotic symptoms. She was high energy; I never saw anything psychotic in her personality.

"You're just on the Depakote then?"

"Yup. And I've been just fine."

This was right after Thanksgiving. When it seemed that we'd settled the medication issue, I launched into my usual questions about what her days were like, what she did with her time, who she lived with, what was important to her. With that, she sprang to life and launched into a long discourse on gravy. She'd just made gravy for that Thanksgiving dinner and she gave me the full description. She always had a helper with her, whose job it was to be the taster.

"I line up ten little spoons on the counter." With each new ingredient, her helper would use a new spoon for another sample.

The next time we met she told me about her stained glass projects. They were elaborate works of art, lost when she'd moved out of the home she'd shared with her husband. I never heard why that marriage ended or how she wound up as one of our clients. Gracie told me she had called social services one day and said, "Get me out of here," and they got her out of there. With Gracie, you didn't get a lot of explanation.

A few months into our work together, Jamal let me know that Gracie had crashed. She had lost her usual equanimity and ended up in a huge fight with her roommates.

Gracie was outraged and demanded that Jamal find her a new place to live. "So I took her around and showed her the options," he said. "A couple of board and care homes that had openings."

He didn't have to say any more, to me or to Gracie. She made amends with her housemates, and they let her stay.

The board and care homes I'd seen were clean and well-kept, but the residents were isolated from one another in their own capsules of loathing and distrust. No one seemed to form friendships or play games or converse with their fellow residents. People took walks but they walked alone.

The kitchens are always off-limits and the house managers provide meals. They are the only ones allowed in the kitchens. A more meaningless life could not be designed if you tried. There are a few exceptions, but they are rare.

When I was in my last month at the clinic and had told a few people that I was leaving, word got around among my patients. One day Gracie exploded into my office to express herself.

"Can't we nail you to the floor here? You can't leave."

"I know," I said. "It's not great for anyone."

In that moment I felt terrible about it. I'd handed in my resignation months ago, trusting that my boss would find someone to take my place in plenty of time for the next doctor to overlap with me. I pictured a warm handoff with each of my patients, a quick introduction before I left. I counted on having the time to train my replacement, as Sophie had done with me.

But nobody had come. And three months later, there was still no one to replace me. I had had a caseload of more than a hundred patients, some of whom I never even met. All of those would be parceled out among the remaining psychiatrists. One of these was two days a week. Another was Dr. Wilson, who was often absent. A third was lending a hand one day a week. He was off-site, always described as "back there," somewhere behind our building, I guessed.

Nobody wanted to come and work with us. Psychiatrists are scarce these days. We occupy a unique niche, being MDs and also trained to do psychotherapy. There's been a shortage of psychiatrists since the '90s, and a job like this one is not attractive. The pay is low, the location unattractive, and the patient population is challenging.

Just as I was preparing to leave, our wonderful nurse, Angela, left too. She told us the county would not hire her on a permanent basis but had strung her along for years as a locum tenens (paid by the hour). I was a locum, too. It's cheaper for the county, since it doesn't have to pay benefits or sick pay, and it can terminate the employee at will, at any time, with no reason given.

The last time I met with Gracie she was settled again with her roommates, in her old routine. It felt very sad saying goodbye, but Gracie didn't let things get heavy. She launched into an account of oil painting on tiny canvases. She didn't mention the uproar with her roommates, the days when she'd gone off the rails and nearly lost her home. I didn't mention it either.

When time was running out, it felt strange not to make a return appointment, and we remarked on that. We stood together, facing each other, wondering how to conclude this last meeting, I guess. I towered over her, although I'm not tall.

I had fretted the previous fall about Gracie, who vaped with abandon and had a disturbing cough. She sounded like she had fluid in her lungs. She sounded short of breath when she spoke. Something evil was growing in her lungs, I was sure. I'd gone around and around with her about getting the chest X-ray that had been ordered, sooner rather than later.

But Gracie wouldn't do it sooner. She was putting it off until later, so she could combine the $5 bus ride with another errand. Now it was the end of March, and she was better. Stronger, not short of breath. She ignored the advice, and it was fine. Gracie had amazing strength.

It felt horrible to be saying goodbye, and I did what I'd do with a friend. I folded her skeletal shoulders in a hug and we embraced.

But as she was about to walk out the door, she turned back. "Could you write me another prescription for the Seroquel, just in case?"

Seroquel is what you take when you feel you're losing it. When the regular mood stabilizer isn't keeping you stable. We'd tried just the Depakote, and clearly that wasn't enough. It was the closest Gracie came to mentioning her awful fight with her roommates.

The Crucial Role of Families

LISTEN TO THE FAMILIES

As a psychiatrist caring for patients with severe mental illness, I find that family involvement often makes the difference between treatment success or treatment failure—and often the difference between life and death for their afflicted loved ones. Family members are the ones who know my patients best. Often the parents have struggled for years to get help for their sons and daughters, petitioning the public guardian, judges, social workers, hospital authorities, and others in heroic efforts to get help, usually with scant success. Tragically they are forced to watch as their once-promising sons and daughters deteriorate for lack of care.

In California, parents are often excluded from discussions of their children's treatment, although they are the ones with the most intimate knowledge of their children's lives. Often they are excluded from writ hearings, which are conducted at the hospital for the purpose of challenging the 5150 hold and discharging the patient, usually successful.

Although parents often provide food and shelter for their grown children after they leave the hospital, they are not only excluded from writ hearings, but they are not even notified when their children leave the hospital. Their grown children, still acutely ill, are often discharged to the street with no follow-up plan for care.

It doesn't have to be this way. In Pennsylvania, for example, a far more humane and effective system involves families from the outset. For an account of the Pennsylvania system and the stark contrast with the

California system, read Jason Park's account of his hospitalization for bipolar disorder in both states (Park, 2023).

Families are our patients' best advocates. For the sake of our patients who suffer from severe mental illness, we need to listen to their families.

Two Houses

Cassandra, who was almost 40 when I met her, spent most of her days with her mother. On her quiet days, she clung to her as they ran errands around town. Other days she wasn't so quiet. On a recent trip to the bank, Cassandra had treated the whole room to a loud, expletive-filled harangue. All business stopped and heads turned to gawk as Cassandra's mother took her by the arm and gently towed her out to the street, her daughter still shrieking at the stunned crowd behind them.

On this day, Cassandra and her mom sat at my desk and talked in tandem. Cassandra spoke in bursts, her speech strangely unmodulated but urgent. Her mother waited for a pause and then leaned forward and quietly updated me on how her daughter was doing. "It's been rough," she said. "She won't go anywhere. She thinks people are talking about her behind her back. Even the store down the street—they know us, they *like* her. She won't go in."

"Mom, you know they're talking about me. I hear them. They talk about my sex life. They say I smell."

"Cassie." Her mom sighed. "No one is talking about you."

When Cassandra went across the hall to the nurse's office, I asked her mom if things were getting worse.

"No, not really. Just one of those bad patches."

I heard this with relief. If Cassandra had become even more ill, we needed to rethink our treatment plan. She'd already been through a few different drug cocktails, and this one seemed to be the best we could find. After they left, I would renew Cassandra's medications.

Officially, this was a medication check for Cassandra. But more important was the chance for Cassandra's mom to talk. My job was to bear witness.

Cassandra and her father had quarreled long ago, when she first became ill in her early twenties. Any argument that she was "sick" made no sense to him. Unable to bear her irrational rages, he moved out of the house into an apartment. But the parents missed each other. In the beginning, Cassandra's mom would make hurried visits to see her husband, then return to spend the night with her fearful daughter.

By this point, though, Cassandra had the family home to herself at night. It was a big house for one person. But she'd been a grown-up for two decades. She could spend the night alone in her childhood home with her mother nearby, just a phone call away in case of emergency. And her mother spent nights with her husband again. This was the bargain the parents made with their fate. The family home for peace. The mother's life for her daughter.

At the end of the hour, Cassandra was still wild and fearful. Her mother, with all the restraint her daughter lacked, put on her coat and stood to leave without my calling time. *She doesn't want to take too much*, I thought to myself. Her loneliness and despair washed over me as I watched her, and I found myself making unnecessary chitchat in a vain effort to cheer her up.

FOUND AND LOST: AMARI

Amari's mother brought him to all his clinic appointments, although by the time I met him he was 28. The first time they came to my office it was October, just before Halloween. A few of the case managers were already wearing bits of Halloween costume.

Amari sat against the back wall, as far away from me as he could get. He was dressed in baggy sweatpants and a hoodie with the drawstring cinched tight, showing only a small oval of his face. As we talked, he kept his head down, as if to make sure I didn't call on him to speak.

It was his mother, Sara, who sat at my desk and did the talking. She spoke quietly as she stated the obvious. "Amari's not doing well." She spoke about his leaving his board and care home to live on the streets, riding the bus for shelter. She mentioned that he'd been off his medication for weeks now.

Amari kept his eyes on the floor, and it seemed as if he was trying to fade into the wall. I imagined he was being assailed by auditory hallucinations—voices ridiculing him and warning him to stay quiet. The voices our patients hear are often cruel and demeaning, even threatening. They are rarely pleasant and often put into words the person's worst fears and most shameful beliefs about themselves. These beliefs in turn are often delusional versions of themselves. Such hostile self-torture is common in schizophrenia.

"Do you want to add anything, Amari?" I asked. I knew he wouldn't, but I didn't want to talk about him as if he wasn't there. He shook his head, not looking up.

Three days after that first visit, Sara left an urgent message on my voicemail. "Amari left his board and care home the day we saw you. Nobody's seen him since." She'd filed a missing person report with the police.

I caught up with his case manager, Malik, who shrugged when I told him about Sara's call. "She's been calling me, too," he said. "Amari *always* comes back." He turned away then, clearly ready to be done with this conversation.

Malik was muscle-bound with a shaved head. His office was at the other end of the clinic from mine, and we saw each other from across the room at team meetings but rarely spoke.

I called Sara to see if Amari was back.

"No. His grandmother caught sight of him in Richmond. She said he didn't look good." Her tone was even, as if holding herself back from yelling at me. I hung up the phone, feeling heavy with foreboding.

As the days went by, Sara left me more messages. Amari's uncle saw him one day and tried to talk to him, but his nephew fled. As soon as she got that call, Sara drove to where her son had been seen, then up and down every street in the neighborhood, but he was gone. His uncle left food out for him and a jacket in case he came back. By then it was mid-November, and the weather had turned cold.

I tried to reach Malik to see if he could help. He'd been Amari's case manager for the past nine years, and I assumed he knew Amari far better than I did. The case manager's job is to get their clients into housing and on "benefits," meaning SSI disability payments and health insurance, usually Medi-Cal. Beyond that, they are expected to bring their clients to medical appointments as needed, including their appointments at our clinic, with the psychiatrist and the nurse. But it was only Amari's mother who ever brought him to see us.

Malik was nowhere to be found. I assumed he was out seeing clients in the field and tried to reach him on both of his cell phones, the county phone and his personal phone, but he never answered. As time went on, I got the feeling that Malik resented having to do this job. It's difficult work, and he'd been there for the last nine years, at least. He needed a new job.

When I mentioned my worry about Amari to Dorothy, the receptionist I knew best, she said, "Who's his case manager?"

"Malik," I said.

She rolled her eyes.

If this were 50 years ago, I would have found a hospital bed for Amari, as he was too overwhelmed by psychosis to be treated in the clinic. I would have seen him every day in the hospital and worked with him to understand what was going on in his life and to find the right medication for him at the right dose. I would have met with his mother. Most likely, he would have left the hospital relieved of his paralyzing psychosis. But today almost all our psychiatric hospitals have been shut down. Today there are so few hospital beds that a threat of imminent violence is often required for hospital admission. People who formerly would have received hospital treatment are treated today in the jails and prisons, which have taken over nearly all our inpatient psychiatric care.

Amari spent most of his time living like a homeless person, camped out on a BART train or an AC Transit bus. If it weren't for his mom, Amari probably would have joined the thousands of homeless souls who live permanently on our streets today. What began as a trickle of street people when the state hospitals began to shut down fifty years ago is now an ocean of misery. People too sick to use treatment and social services survive by foraging in garbage cans. I wondered if Amari was doing that too.

After seventeen days, Amari's bus pass ran out and he called his mom. When they came back to see me, Amari sat as before with his back against the far wall, his thin body wrapped in baggy sweatpants and a hoodie drawn protectively around his face. When I spoke to him, he answered in faint half-words.

Sara said she was keeping her wandering son close by her side, back at the family home since he'd called her. When he went across the hall to the nurse's office, I asked her why he couldn't just live at his own home, instead of the board and care home.

She looked stricken. "When he first got sick, he began to punch walls," she said. "Then he began to punch his brother and sister. He couldn't live at home anymore."

I thought about the terrible dilemma facing parents whose children develop a psychotic illness. Although medication with a good early intervention program can reverse the downward course of the illness, those programs are extremely scarce and insurance balks at paying for them. In the meantime, parents rely on the inadequate care left after the hospitals were shut down.

Amari was supposed to be living at a board and care home, where the board and care operator was supposed to give him his daily medication. But Amari never stayed at that home for more than a day before wandering off. Even if he had stayed, board and care operators have to be skilled and highly motivated in order to oversee their clients' medication. They're not trained healthcare professionals. Most are simply homeowners who've turned their old houses into board and care homes. They're overwhelmed with the job of providing three meals a day and a clean house for their residents.

And so the parents watch helplessly as their sons and daughters grow sicker and end up living on the street, if not in jail.

Amari did return to his board and care home but left again after a day. This time the police found him and took him to John George, the county psychiatric hospital, where he stayed for a week. A week at John George is like winning the lottery. Amari must have impressed the ER doctor with his devastating psychosis, enough to gain admission to the hospital.

The next time I saw Amari and his mother was just before Christmas. This time it was Amari who sat across from me at my desk while his mom stayed in the background. He was dressed in a T-shirt and jeans, and he looked straight at me and began to speak as soon as we sat down.

"I'm bored. There's nothing to do."

I couldn't help smiling. "You're looking great."

"I guess. But I'm bored."

I was still getting used to this new Amari. He might be able to work, I thought, or go to school. "We could get you started with Crystal in voc rehab."

"Hook me up."

The psychiatrist at John George had stopped all Amari's old medications. Then he started him on Haldol, an old-fashioned, inexpensive antipsychotic drug. Amari agreed to take a monthly injection of Haldol as well as the Haldol tablets. Although Haldol can cause muscle spasms, and we often give another drug to forestall that side effect, Amari was one of the people who don't suffer those ill effects. It was exactly the right medication for him.

Amari's on course for a good life, I thought. It's rare to see such a transformation in one of our patients and wonderful. I left that meeting buoyant with hope.

In January, when Amari's mom called to cancel his appointment, I assumed it was because he was doing so well. He wouldn't need new prescriptions for another couple of months, and I wasn't worried. I knew Sara had other children, too. Her daughter was applying to college, and Sara was taking her around the country to visit college campuses. I was on vacation for most of February, so we rescheduled for March. But then Amari again failed to make his appointment.

I was disappointed but also buried in work, and I didn't investigate. With more than a hundred patients in my caseload, I was still seeing some for the first time and fitting others into my schedule at the last minute when their case managers asked, always because it had been way too long since they'd seen a psychiatrist.

Two weeks later, Malik sent me a terse email: "Amari's hearing voices. Needs relief. Walked up to John George six times, they won't take him."

John George, the county hospital, was where Amari had gotten help. Of course he went back there, trusting that John George would take him in again. But although he was clearly suffering, Amari was always refused admission. Evidently the hospital was so crowded that you only got one chance.

Alarmed, I called his mother and got no answer. In fact, although I continued to call, I never did reach her and never saw Amari again. In the meantime, I struggled to understand what had happened, hoping there was something I could do.

I wondered if Amari had been getting his monthly injections of Haldol and went to the nurse's office to check. She showed me two doses of injectable Haldol, the two he should have gotten since Christmas. Case managers are supposed to bring their clients to the clinic for injections, but Malik never did that. For Amari, there was only his mother.

If Malik and I had diligently collaborated on Amari's care, we would have noticed that both Amari's mother and I would be away in February, and Amari would need someone else to make sure he got his medication. But we never had that discussion.

I checked the computer to make sure he was still getting all his oral medications. I scrolled through RxNT, the program we and the pharmacies use to manage prescriptions, and saw that the Haldol, which had been so helpful, had been stopped. In its place was a hefty dose of Seroquel XR, a slow-release drug that often keeps people sedated, day and night. I was horrified. Amari must have hated it. He probably refused it after the first dose.

I saw it had been a year since he'd taken the Seroquel, long before I met him, and then only briefly. Obviously it hadn't helped him. I was appalled and couldn't understand why he was back on it.

Then I remembered that pharmacies could charge $15 a day for Seroquel XR, while Haldol was only 50 cents a day. Our clinic operation was often chaotic, but the business of selling drugs hums along efficiently. It is perfectly legal for the pharmacy staff to call for a refill of any prescription on record for the patient. They can request a refill of the medication that looks the most up to date, but they can also request a refill of any drug that hasn't been discontinued by the prescriber.

Since the pharmacies deliver medication directly to the board and care homes, out of sight of the prescriber, no one keeps tabs on their choices. The only way to prevent the switch to a long-discontinued drug is for us, the prescribers, to laboriously retrace the patient's prescription history in the computer and write "discontinue" on each outdated prescription. We don't always do that, and until just then, I hadn't realized we needed to.

Meanwhile, on the first possible date, the pharmacy's automated system sends out refill requests, creating a chaotic pile of faxes for us prescribers. We were so thinly staffed that we might hastily okay a refill for a patient whose regular doctor was away. If we didn't respond to a fax, the pharmacy would make an urgent call. In my experience, the caller was always a woman, sounding young and vulnerable.

"Amari needs a refill on his Seroquel," she would have said. "He's running out!"

Then my tired colleague must have obliged, and a long-dead prescription came back to life, a pharmaceutical Frankenstein.

MELA SHALIMAR

Meeting with Aminah was always a group affair. When my colleagues at the clinic saw all the chairs gathered in my office, they'd smile. "Looks like you had a party in here!"

It never felt like a party. Five of us—Aminah's case manager, the Punjabi interpreter, Aminah and her husband, Tarik, and I would gather in a tense group around my desk. The interpreter, a quiet woman with a gentle smile, sat next to Aminah as if to steady her. It was clear that under the polite surface a battle raged between husband and wife. Tarik always prevailed, leaving Aminah vanquished and fuming. It was at his insistence that Aminah was in treatment.

They came from the city of Lahore in Pakistan, first Tarik and his brother, who settled in Fremont and built a small business. After they'd established a beachhead in America, Tarik brought Aminah and their young son to join him. But while the brothers thrived in California, Aminah never learned English.

No one had seen this coming. Back in Lahore, she had finished college with honors. But here Aminah became strange and wandered the neighborhood, talking to herself.

Tarik was mortified. He tried to keep her at home. Aminah filed for divorce. Tarik went to court and halted the proceedings. Aminah feared Tarik was plotting to poison her. At home she talked to herself when she thought no one noticed. Out of desperation, Tarik brought her to our clinic for help.

My predecessor, Sophie, had started her on Risperdal, a modern antipsychotic drug. Aminah seemed calmer but she complained it made her feel groggy and, worse, it was making her fat. Then Sophie left and I became Aminah's doctor.

Aminah wanted to stop the Risperdal, whereas Tarik wanted her on the maximum dose. It took time, over repeated clinic visits, for me and Aminah, with Tarik anxiously protesting, to work out the right dosage. The conversation was always cumbersome, as all the back and forth between me and Aminah had to go through the interpreter. And there were constant interruptions by Tarik and furious side conversations in Punjabi between Tarik and Aminah.

Aminah's case manager, Tony, was a silent presence. He seemed impatient for us to finish our medication talk so he could get on with his agenda. He had forms to fill out for benefits for banking, housing, and schooling. Each item needed to be checked off his list each time.

Tony was dedicated and tireless in his attention to detail. He had been a parole officer before moving on to social work and carried a vaguely menacing aura. He had a buzz cut, huge arms, and heavy shoulders. He ran our meetings with iron efficiency.

One day, after we had finally settled on the right dose of medication and Aminah seemed happier than I'd ever seen her, I steeled myself and let them know I was leaving the clinic. I had handed in my resignation, and I told them our next meeting would be my last. Aminah and Tarik seemed shocked, and I felt my sadness and regret well up in me all over again. Then we all looked at our calendars to set up that last meeting.

The date we found happened to fall on a major holiday in Lahore—the Festival of Lights. When we set the date, the Pakistanis lit up and told us Americans about the coincidence. Tony let it pass, but I made a note of it.

When the day arrived, I received an email message from Tony. "Detained for emergency. Translator engaged. Go ahead without me."

So it was just the four of us—Tarik and Aminah, the translator, and me. Meeting without Tony's steely presence felt like a school holiday. "Happy Festival of Lights!" I said, and everyone smiled. It sounded silly in English, I guess, but that day I didn't care.

"What do you call it in your own language?"

The translator smiled gently. "Mela Shalimar."

Later I learned that the holiday commemorated a 16th-century Sufi saint who had lived in Lahore. The festival was first held in the Shalimar Gardens just outside the city.

"How do you celebrate it?"

Tarik sat forward with his phone, tapped the screen, and handed it to me. "It's been outlawed now, but we have an underground channel."

I glanced at the interpreter. "Outlawed?"

She shrugged and half nodded.

I took the phone and saw a village of red stone. The last light was fading from the sky and men in white robes and turbans wound through the streets in a long parade, each one with a flaming torch held aloft. They seemed to come from far away, tiny figures in the distance growing larger as they approached, then smaller again till they disappeared from view.

It was a movie, and I watched the screen, mesmerized. Right there in my windowless office with its blank white walls, plastic chairs, and government-issue calendar, I traveled with the Pakistanis across the world and back in time to old Lahore to see the Festival of Lights.

A MOTHERLESS SOLDIER

Sadie was an army vet back from Afghanistan, discharged early with post-traumatic stress disorder. I was her new doctor at Dry Valley. Her medical record told me nothing, so I filled in the gaps. I imagined her as tall and powerful, a modern-day Amazon. Instead, Sadie was short and neatly dressed, her face carefully made up. She wore her hair in a medium

Afro and smiled shyly as I introduced myself. She was young enough to be my daughter. I couldn't picture her as a soldier.

She said nothing about the war and talked only about her mother. "When I went to Afghanistan, I couldn't take care of my mom anymore, so we put her in a home." Her voice shook and she stopped.

Her sadness flooded through me, and I wanted to be comforting, but Sadie was working to steady herself, so I stayed quiet.

"As soon as I got home, I went to see her. She's changed."

Each time Sadie came to see me, she started with a report on her mother. As I got to know her better, her soldierly qualities revealed themselves. She was stoic now, almost matter of fact as she relayed the news.

"My mom's losing her memory," she said one day.

A month later, "She can't remember my name."

Sadie didn't brag about her service, but I was curious. I wanted to know what she did over there.

"I drove a truck," she said. I imagined her driving an army truck along those booby-trapped roads, waiting for a roadside IED to explode and blow her to pieces. Sadie never elaborated and I didn't want to push her. But finally I thought to ask what she transported in the truck.

"Tanks," she said. "It was a flatbed truck." It was a huge truck, with an armored tank secured to its enormous bed. It was a challenge to maneuver and Sadie bumped into things.

"What kind of things?" I asked, fearing injuries, loss of life.

"A gatepost and some fencing," she said. "It was a narrow gate. You had to aim the truck just right to get through it." Those accidents undid her. All that terror she must have kept in check, day after day, waiting for the bomb to go off. Until at the end, all it took was a flattened fence, and she collapsed.

Sadie was still waiting for the bomb to explode, except this time it would be the loss of her mother. One day, it happened.

"She doesn't even recognize me," she said with a wail of desperation. Then her voice turned hard. "I blame God. I go to church every Sunday. And God lets this happen to me?" She gave away all her church clothes, swearing she was done with God.

Sadie lived in a board and care home on a tiny disability allowance. She had no friends there. Her brothers didn't see her, and she made no effort to contact them. Instead, she spent all her time behind the house, shooting hoops.

After we'd been meeting for a few months, she changed her mind about church. "But first I need church clothes," she said. Neither of us mentioned that she gave the old ones away. Now the problem was financial. It would take time to save up her meager disability pay.

In the meantime, she kept shooting hoops.

"You must be very good by now," I said one day.

That got me a rare smile.

At our Christmas party a month later, I learned why. Every year at Christmastime, the clinic staff puts on a holiday party for all our clients. The large back hall was turned into a Christmas carnival. The conference room became a disco, with Jamal serving as DJ. A disco ball hung from the ceiling in the darkened room. I joined the spectators—patients and staff—who lined the walls and watched the dancers. It was just a few brave souls from vocational rehab who got out in the middle of the room and danced. I watched for a while with admiration and a bit of envy.

In the spacious back hall, the lights were on, and the Good Hope crew had set up games. There was a wooden frame for beanbag toss, and I walked by it quickly. But Sadie was standing there, smiling and waving me back.

"Come on, Dr. Feller!" She held out a beanbag. "You try it!"

I knew I was going to make a fool of myself, but I took the beanbag. A small crowd gathered to watch.

With expert grace Sadie lobbed each bag through the hole. I was even worse than I feared. Some of my beanbags landed on the wooden frame, but others landed ignominiously on the floor beside it. Sadie was kind enough not to laugh but she was ebullient.

I shook my head at how bad I was, but I was smiling. Sadie looked so happy, I couldn't help it.

Across the hall were tables spread with Christmas cookies, brownies, and jugs of mulled cider. But I passed them in a daze, remembering a long-ago summer afternoon when my daughter Jessica was in grade school. We were at the pool with her friend Katie, playing shark and minnow. I was always the hungry shark, forever trying and failing to catch the minnows, who dodged out of my reach with joyful shrieks just as I was about to eat them. We played that game all summer.

LEAVING DRY VALLEY: GEORGE AND LUTHER

At Dry Valley, I noticed that the people who do unusually well in spite of their dire illnesses tend to be the ones with strong family connections: mothers or fathers who hang in there, siblings who stay in touch, and sometimes their own children whom they care for. Since then, I've met so many mothers whose lives are dominated by their struggles to stay in touch with their severely ill sons and daughters that I realize maintaining a strong connection takes far more than just hanging in there. It seems to me that often it's a matter of luck today: the good fortune not to fall through the cracks of our creaky, broken system and to receive adequate treatment and then to respond well to treatment.

George and his family were lucky on both counts. George lived with his two kids, a couple of nephews, and his mother, who kept the household going. Without her, he might have lost his kids. But his mother was old, and he worried. His voices harped on this fear. "Your mother's going to die," they'd say.

George suffered from diabetes as well as schizophrenia. Already he'd lost sensation in one of his feet due to diabetic neuropathy. His circulation was poor, and he didn't heal well. He knew that a small injury to that foot could lead to amputation. The voices seized on this fear, too. "Your leg's going to fall off," they'd say.

George spent hours every day helping his children with their homework. I always asked after his kids, to see the look of pride on his face.

This day he said, "My older boy is getting all A's." He beamed, then his face sagged a little. "Except for Mandarin—"

"Mandarin?" It seemed a bit much for grade school.

He nodded and then we laughed together.

We talked a little more and he said, "I'm 90% normal. The neighbors don't know there's anything wrong with me."

"How do you do it?"

He considered. "I see you. I get my injections every month. And I pray. Every night, for half an hour, I pray."

Then there was Luther. He seemed so normal, I wondered if his only problem was binge drinking, now in the past. That was the way he remembered it. I wondered if we were giving him drugs he didn't need.

So one day I did a deep dive into his history. His electronic medical record didn't give much detail, but it did list the county agencies that provided care for him. Occasionally there were clinical details. I scrolled through the years. Every county mental health service was listed, back to when he was 18. Santa Rita, John George, a few outpatient clinics, and one stay at Sierra.

I'd hoped it was all a big mistake, that he was really just an alcoholic misdiagnosed with schizophrenia. I liked this guy a lot. But it turned out that he was not misdiagnosed. He wasn't always this normal; he'd had episodes of psychosis with paranoid delusions. It wasn't just alcohol.

At team meeting, vocational rehab reported Luther was failing on his job because he didn't smile enough. We were outraged on his behalf. Smiling was not his thing; he had a dry sense of humor. So the voc rehab counselor found him a night job sweeping floors. Smiling wouldn't be an issue there.

Luther lived in a board and care home but, like George, he had a car and a driver's license. And a family. He saw his brothers and sisters on a regular basis and always had, throughout his illness. His sister left one of her windows unlocked for him, day and night, even when she was out of town, so Luther could always go to her house if he was locked out at night. Now that he was working nights, the board and care home was giving him grief about his late hours. Board and care homes are not designed for people who work.

The last time I saw Luther, I told him that I was leaving and was sorry I hadn't told him earlier. He said he'd heard.

We talked a bit and then I asked about his drinking. "How's it going with the alcohol?"

"I've had two beers in the last two months," he said. "I walked out of the store and drank them both. Then a cop came along." He paused.

"What happened?"

"He said, 'You've been drinking.' I said, 'Yes I have.'" Another pause.

"What happened then?" I asked.

"He went one way, and I went the other way."

I smiled. I would miss him, his dry humor and understated manner. I wanted to tinker with something, adjust some medication, do some test, just to give me a reason to bring him back one more time. But there wasn't really anything to do.

Luther looked up at the faded Picasso print on my office wall above the cupboard.

"Is that a Picasso?"

"A really faded Picasso," I said.

"We used to play this game in my family called The Great Artists." He knew the painting.

We talked about it a little more, how washed out the oranges and blues looked. Then it felt too painful to go on, so I said we'd better stop.

Luther's not the kind of guy you hug goodbye. I closed the door behind him and sat there stunned. It took me a while to collect myself and get back to work. It wasn't just Luther. It was everyone I was leaving behind.

CHAPTER 12

Living on the Edge in the 21st Century

FULL-SERVICE PARTNERSHIP

After leaving Dry Valley, I took a job at a mental health agency, in its "full-service partnership" (FSP). The FSP was tasked with caring for the city's most disabled by severe mental illness. Its mission was to provide a comprehensive and intensive mental health program for adults with severe and persistent mental illness. FSPs are often known as "hospitals without walls," although, in reality, they do not provide what a hospital does.

The FSP was staffed by a team of social workers who enrolled clients on disability insurance and Medi-Cal and tried to find housing for them. The agency's nursing staff helped out with the clients' medical problems. But when my boss showed me around my first day on the job, he said, "I never know what to do with a psychiatrist on the FSP." Although our clients suffered from severe mental illness, it had been a year since the team had a psychiatrist. After I left, the FSP team would go another year without a psychiatrist. I came to believe that for this FSP, the mission was to provide social services for our clients but that psychiatric care was not an important part of the mission.

On paper, I had a large caseload but most of my patients were ghosts, mere rumors. I read their scanty notes in the electronic medical record (EMR) and imagined them but I never saw them. The homeless man who bedded down by the bay, for example, and another man who camped near the mouth of a tunnel. Both were scheduled to meet with me one afternoon, and I read about them in the EMR, hoping to see them. But neither one could be found. I had too many no-shows, too much empty space in my schedule. It was demoralizing.

As time went on, I sensed that many of us on the FSP team also struggled with a sense of futility. We tried to help our desperately needy clients when we saw them. But the first battle was simply to see them. Finding them was often a hopeless pursuit.

In team meeting, the case managers sped through their roster of clients. Mostly they reported in monosyllables, which I gathered meant "status quo." Often the report just recounted a failed search.

"The door was open, I called his name—nothing. I didn't think I should go in."

"You can bill for the trip out there," the team leader told him.

The air felt heavy with failure.

Then one day we had a visit from the homeless outreach and treatment team (HOTT), whose job it was to connect with people living on the street and then to introduce them to us. The HOTT team leader, a willowy man with a shock of pink hair, arrived in high spirits to tell us about Emmylou. "I guarantee she'll be your favorite client," he told us.

Emmylou was an elegant street person who treated herself to a high level of hygiene. She rigged up an outdoor shower, screened by a hanging curtain for modesty. She decorated her little tent with colored ribbons tied to the tentpole. Already she'd visited our clinic and met Marina, our security officer. Emmylou's main concern was for her stuff, which she'd have to leave outside in her shopping cart. But Marina promised to keep an eye on it. So Emmylou said she would return for services. The HOTT team leader left a ripple of quiet excitement in his wake.

When the day came, though, Emmylou had vanished. Her tent was in its usual place in the park, and her shopping cart sat next to the tent. Her would-be case manager, the one from the FSP, searched the entire park and the streets around it as well, but she was gone.

It seemed the people we wanted to serve didn't always value our services. We had to lure them in. The best lure we had was money. Once the clients agreed to accept services, the case manager could sign them up for benefits, including Social Security disability. If the client was unable to manage their own funds (true of almost all our clients), the case manager became the designated representative payee (Social Security Administration, n.d.). Designation as the representative payee for clients is a powerful tool for the case manager, who sets up savings accounts for their clients, manages their funds, and issues checks as appropriate. Our clients were often reluctant to come to the clinic, but usually met with their case managers in order to pick up their checks.

Money was a constant concern for my boss, who often confided in me about his money worries. I wondered why he'd hired me, worried as he was about money. Then one day he told me the city had taken the representative payee function away from our clinic and given it to another agency, which would hand out the checks. However, he said, our agency would pay the other agency to perform this service.

We had an all-staff meeting to discuss how we might lure the clients back to the clinic once we no longer had checks to give them. Someone suggested coupons, redeemable at the corner store, as a reward for coming in to see us. We couldn't pay the clients directly, but we could pay the corner store. It was the best plan anyone could think of.

SLEEPING ROUGH

By the time we reached Mr. Van Dyke's campsite under the freeway, it was midafternoon. He and his partner lay in their sleeping bags, watching as we approached. The heavy gray concrete overpass kept the site dry, but the air was chilled, even on that warm summer day. Their bags lay in the dirt, surrounded by fast food wrappers, empty cracker boxes, and a menagerie of dusty stuffed animals. At their feet, a swivel chair tilted sideways, its wheels sunk into the loose ground.

I had ridden to the site with Isaac, Mr. Van Dyke's caseworker. His mission that day was to persuade the couple to move into a hotel. Our agency would pick up the tab.

Sharon, our nurse, was already at the site. Her mission was to change the dressing on Mr. Van Dyke's open wound, no small feat under those conditions. But she was waiting for us, the dressing change already done when we arrived. Isaac nodded at me to start my interview with Mr. Van Dyke.

I introduced myself and squatted on the ground at his side, but he turned away. His thinning hair fell in long dirty strands around his neck. Everything I said he greeted with a wall of silence. His partner smiled kindly at me, and I saw she was missing a few of her front teeth.

Finally I asked, "When was the last time you slept indoors?"

At that, he turned on me, his voice a scream of fury. "The last time I let the FSP put me in a hotel, they stole my stuff. All of it. Even my log." He stabbed a ballpoint pen at a spiral notebook beside him, open to a page half filled with writing. "See this? My log. They take all my shit, every time."

I studied the log, glad of this small opening.

Isaac edged forward then, signaling my time was up. We'd spoken for less than five minutes. Clients who are sick enough to be in our program are required to be seen periodically by a psychiatrist. This would be it for Mr. Van Dyke, unless something extraordinary happened.

As soon as I was back in my office, I pulled up his record in the EMR to record my visit and to learn what I could about Mr. Van Dyke. His diagnosis in the EMR was schizophrenia. I expected it would be. Every one of our patients is labeled with the most severe mental illness possible, almost always schizophrenia. It's called "up-coding." It's harder to deny payment for severe psychosis than for, say, depression. A primary diagnosis of substance abuse excludes the patient from all payment.

"Just ignore it," my boss told me when I remarked on the uniformity of our clients' diagnoses. "The caseworkers put that in. Just make your own diagnosis."

I certainly would make my own diagnosis, but I couldn't change the initial diagnosis in the EMR. It was assigned at intake and locked in. I understood this system was strictly for billing purposes, but it wasn't something I could discuss with my boss. We didn't deal in those kinds of truths.

Mr. Van Dyke didn't seem as if he could be schizophrenic, although what he'd told me sounded delusional. But I was impressed that he had a steady partner, which was rare for someone with untreated schizophrenia. Based on the empty junk food wrappers, his delusional rage, and his partner's missing front teeth, I wondered if Mr. Van Dyke and his partner both had a methamphetamine problem. That would be good news if we were planning to treat Mr. Van Dyke, because addiction is challenging but treatable. With good care and steady effort, he could overcome an addiction and make a full return to normal life. But we weren't talking about treatment. We were just talking about how to move him into a hotel.

In the team meeting that morning, Isaak noted that Mr. Van Dyke was camped out with his partner, who would be helpful in the effort to move the couple into a hotel, a move that he was resisting. Although our agency was listed as a mental health service, our largest single expense in past years had been for the "respite" program, which paid for temporarily housing people who were living on the street in hotels. I assumed this arrangement was still in place, because in a recent team meeting, we had been warned that our large respite budget was already running out.

There was no plan to treat Mr. Van Dyke for any mental health problem. I was there with Isaak and the nurse that day so the medical record could show that he had been seen by a psychiatrist for his quarterly psychiatry appointment, as required. The regulations mandate this quarterly visit, but there is no way to require that meaningful treatment be provided. For Mr. Van Dyke, that would have meant making regular visits with him and his partner, an assessment of his mental health problem, and a good faith effort to provide adequate treatment.

In my experience at Dry Valley and especially at the FSP, the case managers were dedicated and hardworking but generally saw their mission as separate from the business of combating mental illness. In team meetings, mental illness was rarely mentioned in connection with a client. In general, that topic was confined to the disability forms that caseworkers filled out and brought to me for my signature. Those disability forms detailed the level of impairment but never a specific diagnosis. Certainly our caseworkers appreciated that their clients struggled with mental illness, but understanding the symptoms that disabled our clients was not part of their mission.

By contrast, in a primary care clinic, the entire staff collaborates on treatment because they can talk openly about a patient's reason for coming to the clinic. Perhaps the difference at the FSP and at Dry Valley was the belief that acknowledging mental illness stigmatized the client.

If mental illness and its treatment *had* been a topic of conversation, we would have talked about what it would take to treat Mr. Van Dyke. I would have suggested that I drive out to their encampment under the freeway to talk with him and his partner. It also would have meant that I made my own schedule at the FSP, seeing patients as often as I could and going to their homes (or campsites) on my own if necessary.

For reasons I never understood, the case managers were hesitant to let me visit patients on my own, as with Kerry, who told me he was "homeless by choice."

"HOMELESS BY CHOICE"

When I met Kerry, he'd been living on the streets for years. He was a Vietnam vet. I had several chairs in my office, and he took the one that kept his back to the wall and with a straight line of sight to the door. Briefly I wondered about post-traumatic stress disorder, since he was a combat vet, but he was garrulous and cheerful. He tipped his chair back against the wall and recounted his close calls and courage under fire as an infantryman in Vietnam. He seemed to be enjoying himself.

"I've been homeless by choice since 1965," he told me.

He said it so proudly, I couldn't help myself. "I thought you were in Vietnam in 1965," I said.

"Oh—yeah—1975." He went on unperturbed, expanding on the life of freedom he enjoyed with his friends on the street.

Then Marla, an energetic young social worker, pulled off a coup. She found a one-bedroom apartment for Kerry.

The next time I saw him, he'd moved into his new apartment. All of his bravado was gone that day, and he sat by my desk and stared into the middle distance. He had a haunted look, as if he'd just witnessed a massacre.

"I've got a living room and a kitchen," he said. "And a dining room table."

I asked how it was, having a place indoors.

He shook his head. He still hung out with his friends on the street. "But then at night it's like—'well, see you in the morning'—and I go up to my nice warm bed." He looked miserable. "I can't bring anyone with me or I'll lose the apartment." He fell silent then, staring ahead as if still seeing that wrenching moment when he left his friends huddled on the sidewalk and walked away to his warm bed.

In team meeting a week later, we heard Kerry was still depressed. The problem, Marla said, was that he was isolated. She'd prodded him to go the senior center, where he could have some social activity, but he wouldn't go.

"Could Dr. Feller do a phone interview?" She addressed the room, not me.

I said, "Why couldn't I just go see him?"

She turned to me, and I could see it would be a problem, although I couldn't understand why.

"I can't see him over the phone," I told her.

Marla seemed doubtful but she agreed to meet me at Kerry's new apartment, two blocks away. It was a concrete building, gray and cold. We took the elevator to the third floor and knocked on his door. After some time, Kerry appeared and graciously invited us in. Marla asked me if I was sure I'd be okay without her; if so, she had places to be. Of course I was sure.

The apartment was large, just as he'd said. Furnished, with a big dining room table. Kerry was subdued, a far cry from the jolly old soldier who'd tipped his chair back and told me war stories. He hardly knew how to handle himself; it seemed as if he was overwhelmed by the task of coping with my visit. But he showed me a chair at the big table and took another for himself.

All around us on the floor were new paper bags full of supplies—one from CVS, still stapled shut, another bag with new clothes, another with kitchen supplies. They looked as if they'd been sitting there for a while. He seemed mortified.

"My fault," he said. He should have gotten to it and unpacked. In fact, everything was his fault.

He looked at the unopened pharmacy bag and glanced up at me uneasily. "I know I should have—"

"That's okay. Can I have a look?" Inside were the antidepressants I'd prescribed: a small supply of Zoloft, at Marla's request. He was depressed, but he needed more than pills. I knew he wouldn't take them anyway, because he refused all psych meds.

Weeks later I saw Kerry again, this time much improved. He hadn't touched the Zoloft, he admitted. It was an adventure that morning with his friends on the street that restored his spirits. He still spent his days panhandling with the old crew down on the sidewalk, and on this day, they'd ventured into new territory and upset the neighbors. The police were called, and in the ensuing fracas, he'd been restored to his old place with his friends on the street. He came into my office later that afternoon full of righteous energy, back to his formerly happy self.

I often think of the words spoken by Jesus in the Gospel of Matthew: "Man shall not live by bread alone" (Matt. 4:4, King James Version). He was referring to the need for God, but for me his words call up the human need to belong. Kerry needed his friends on the street as much as he needed food and shelter. Belonging with them gave meaning to his life.

A FATAL OVERDOSE: PATRICK

The worst job I ever had was on the Oakland army base, where I worked for a summer when I was 19. Soldiers on leave from Vietnam would land at all hours, and as soon as they landed they needed their new uniforms, with their new insignia reflecting their new ranks. Accordingly, the army ran an industrial sewing shop on the base where we sewed new insignia onto their jackets and hemmed their pants. To allow the soldiers to get on their way as quickly as possible, the shop ran 24 hours a day. I worked the graveyard shift, from 11:00 p.m. till 8:00 a.m.

We were there for nine hours, but in the middle of the night, we theoretically stopped for lunch, so we got paid for only eight hours. We were supposed to stay awake all night, but no one did. Although it was strictly forbidden, we stretched out on the long sewing tables and slept, waking up to spring into action when another planeload of soldiers landed and a new batch of uniforms was wheeled into the shop. The other women would mob the rack, grabbing armloads of olive drab pants and jackets. They were fast on the machines and whipped through whole stacks of uniforms in the time it took me to finish one. Our base pay was $1.65 an hour, but after that it was piecework.

I was an outsider in that setting, the only one who spoke English. The other women spoke Tagalog, except for our boss, who spoke Japanese. Her English wasn't good enough for her to reprimand me, so she had to settle for glaring at me. I got the distinct feeling that she didn't like me. I was an oddity, a college girl from Berkeley. A hippie with long curly hair and a crash helmet.

The saving grace of that summer was my motorcycle. I rode that bike from Concord to the Oakland army base, 24 miles on the freeway. The best part was going through the Caldecott Tunnel, where the sound of my engine bounced off the concrete walls in a satisfying roar, and the undulations in the pavement gave it a bit of bounce before bursting into the cool night air of Berkeley. It was a joyous moment, that tunnel ride, and it slightly balanced the loneliness I felt at the shop.

When I started work at the FSP, I thought it would be much better than Dry Valley, but it broke my lifetime record for terrible jobs. Come to think of it, my job with the FSP was a bit like that job in the sewing shop. Back then, I was lonely and isolated by language barriers, but also by who I was—a Cal student on summer break. I didn't belong. At the FSP, I was as lonely and isolated as I'd been in that shop, although I struggled to understand why.

I had worked at the FSP for two weeks when Brenda brought Patrick to see me. She stood in the open door of my office with a sour look on her face.

"He's okay to be seen *today*, because he's only a *little* bit drunk. For a change." With that, she was gone. Patrick waited outside my door, a thin, red-faced man who stood looking at his feet.

In staff meetings, I'd been impressed by Brenda's generosity and patience. She seemed to specialize in the impossible clients that other case managers wouldn't touch. When they no-showed for their appointments, she'd go to their homes to see them. When they were kicked out of their board and care homes, she'd shake her head, smile, and find them new homes. I wondered why she was so different with Patrick.

I stood and waved toward the chair beside my desk. "Come on in, Patrick. Have a seat." As he moved by me, I got a whiff of alcohol on his breath, and I waited for him to start, wondering if he'd bring up the topic of his drinking.

To my surprise, he raised his head and looked me in the eye. "I bought a pint this morning," he said, watching me steadily, "but I've been sipping it."

"What do you like to drink?" I'd found long ago that lecturing about the dangers of substance abuse causes instant backtracking, so I aimed for easy and casual. What I wanted was the truth.

"What do I like to drink?" He looked surprised by the question. "Um . . . Jim Beam, usually."

I nodded as if all my patients started their mornings with a pint of bourbon. "So that pint you're sipping this morning—will it last you all day?"

He gave me a look, then shook his head. "Nope. I'll get another later."

I wasn't shocked. I'd had patients who drank a quart a day of hard alcohol every day. "What else? Street drugs?" Usually I had to run through a few possibilities before people felt comfortable telling me about their drug use.

But Patrick didn't hesitate. "Heroin. And fentanyl." He kept his eyes on my face as he spoke. "I've already OD'd once and got rescued. Someone gave me Narcan." He was lucky. Narcan reverses the action of opioid drugs like heroin and fentanyl.

"So next time you might not be so lucky."

"I know." He'd scared himself. It was a rare opening, and we needed to seize the moment. "I'm on the waiting list for Walden House 360," he added.

"The waiting list?" You could die on the waiting list.

"Yes, Brenda's helping me with it."

I'd never heard of Walden House 360, but I assumed it was a chemical dependency program, the best that could be found.

I will always wish that I had buttonholed Brenda that day and asked her about the plan for Patrick. We needed to do better. Something that day, while we had the chance.

But I didn't buttonhole Brenda. The FSP was a rude shock after friendly Dry Valley, where we all had offices together. There we could hang in each other's doors or linger after team meeting and talk. But at the FSP my office was across town from the rest of the team. Although I'd often ridden with case managers to visit clients at Dry Valley, on the FSP the case managers avoided riding with me. It was too bad, because those rides at Dry Valley had been opportunities to make friendly connections, to learn more about the clients we cared for, or just to have pleasant chats.

At the FSP, if the case managers were forced to drive with me to see a client, we rode in awkward silence. Each morning I met with the team, but I learned not to speak in those meetings. If I did, the team leader would cut me off with a weary, "Let's move on." I sensed that all decisions about patient care were strictly up to the case managers. Medical issues were handled between the case managers and the nurses.

The strained atmosphere with the rest of the team was something I'd never experienced before in any medical setting. I tried as hard as I could to be friendly, cooperative, and, above all, respectful. But as time went on, things got worse rather than better. I remember sitting in team meeting one morning and looking around at the others, not one of whom would meet my eyes. It was weird.

If I approached Brenda after team meeting, she turned her back. As I drove across town to my own office, I'd struggle to figure out what I was doing wrong. Later, I decided the team functioned like a wilderness outpost, a tight-knit crew who had each other's backs but resented outsiders. They'd been on their own for a long time, with no psychiatrist, and now they had me plopped into their midst. Occasionally I'd ride with one of the nurses, who tried to be friendly but was clearly looking at me with pity. *She feels bad for me*, I thought.

It seemed that the most respectful thing I could do was to stay in my own lane. It was a narrow lane, as it seemed my job was to renew prescriptions and sign applications for benefits. And see patients as infrequently as possible, so as to avoid making extra work for the case managers, who often had to bring them to my office across town.

Questioning Brenda about her plan for Patrick would have felt like I'd stepped over the line and trespassed into her territory. With Brenda already bristling with disapproval, it might have made things still worse for Patrick, I imagined.

So after Patrick told me of his dire situation, I simply refilled his meds and requested the soonest return appointment with him that I could get. My appointments were set up jointly by the case managers and a couple of clerical workers who sat on the other side of the high wall that divided our office. I would write the desired time frame on a slip of paper and have the client take it to the front window. Someone there would deal with it. But Patrick never appeared on my calendar again.

Perhaps he didn't stop at the window. Perhaps no one was there. Perhaps Brenda didn't want to bring him to my office again.

It was six weeks later when I heard the news. My boss began a meeting with me by announcing that one of my patients had died: Patrick. Nobody knew the cause of death, he said. Then he added that my position was to end in a month. "We're terminating the contract," he said, meaning with the recruiter in Atlanta who'd hired me.

I was stunned. Then everything fell into place. Suddenly I knew why the team members wouldn't meet my eyes, why case managers tried to avoid riding with me, and, if forced to do so, why we rode in awkward silence. Why Sharon, the nurse, looked at me with pity.

"How long has this been in the works?" I asked.

He looked uneasy. "Oh . . . a while."

"Who else are you talking to about it?"

He looked still more guilty. "Not the case managers." Meaning the nurses, who would have passed it on to the case managers immediately. No wonder no one would talk to me or look me in the eye. They were sitting on a secret.

I was so taken aback that I didn't think to ask him why he didn't let me in on this, too. I certainly would have understood, given the FSP's long stretch without any psychiatrist and his constant worry about money.

As soon as he left, I searched for Patrick's treatment record in the EMR, but it was gone. It had been cleared from the system. We had no way to look back at our work and see what we missed. And no one else could see what we missed, either.

But that afternoon, one of our nurses came to see me. "We thought we should provide Narcan to our vulnerable clients," she said. "Because—well, because Patrick . . ." Everyone knew he'd died of an overdose.

Later, when I could stand to think about it, I made some calls. First I called Walden 360, where Patrick had thought he was on the waiting list. No one at Walden 360 ever responded to my many calls and emails. I learned from its website that it offered no services in Alameda County except for an Asian Health Clinic in Fremont. But at Options Recovery, someone answered the phone right away. Options was 20 minutes from our office. It provides housing and long-term treatment for addiction. Newbridge, also close by, runs a residential program with a few beds for people on Medi-Cal. Through Newbridge, I learned Patrick could have gotten medication the day that he first came to see me. He could have gotten methadone or Suboxone. Either would have prevented him from going into heroin withdrawal and bought him time to begin recovery.

And he could have gotten a benzodiazepine, such as Librium or Valium, to prevent complications of alcohol withdrawal, such as delirium tremens (DTs). Clearly he was sipping the bourbon to prevent the onset of alcohol withdrawal, which is painful and sometimes even fatal.

But the bourbon wouldn't prevent heroin withdrawal, so I assumed he would find more heroin soon, to avoid going into opiate withdrawal. Methadone, a long-acting opioid, would have prevented him from going into heroin withdrawal and allowed him to function without nodding out. And it would have been his ticket into residential treatment. It might have saved his life.

Perhaps Brenda had made all these same calls. Perhaps she told Patrick that Walden 360 had nothing for him, and he got confused and thought he was on the waiting list for Walden. But I never asked her. I quit the day I learned of his death, after two months at the FSP.

Chapter 13

Our Broken System

Early Intervention in Schizophrenia

Schizophrenia steals the lives of its victims, often striking before they reach adulthood. Schooling is interrupted, careers are derailed, and social life is upended. Like cancer, it often results in early death from suicide—20 times the usual rate during the first year of illness—and from accidents, drug overdoses, untreated medical illness, and even from police violence (Zaheer, 2020). As with cancer, treatment is not always successful, and relapse is common. But whereas cancer is rightly treated with urgency at the first sign of illness, treatment for schizophrenia is often delayed. As with cancer, putting off treatment is destructive.

People in the first stages of psychosis experience a peculiar unawareness of their illness, termed anosognosia. As Thomas Insel writes in *Healing: Our Path from Mental Illness to Mental Health*, "in many cases the irrationality of psychosis confers a kind of cognitive blindness, complete with a paranoid certainty that everyone else is missing the truth" (Insel, 2022; 149).

The onset of psychosis is terrifying: hallucinations, voices from unseen speakers, often threatening or belittling. Sometimes these voices order acts of violence toward oneself or others. People experience a feeling that their thoughts are leaking out, broadcast to the outside world, with no way to stop them. Just as often, they have a feeling that a foreign presence is directing their thoughts, sometimes by a device placed in the brain. "Brain wave radar," one of my patients called it. Or they feel that strangers are giving them secret signals.

But rather than rush to get medical care, as we might for a suspicious lump, the troubled person feels that other people are causing this suffering. Worried parents, witnessing the odd behavior and personality changes in a son or daughter, start gently, hoping psychotherapy will help. But many therapists have no training or experience with severe mental illness such as schizophrenia. Valuable time is lost trying to treat a brain disorder with psychotherapy only.

It used to be that cancer elicited this same terrified helplessness. It was whispered about, so frightening and misunderstood that people feared that physical contact with the afflicted person would infect them.

Today many forms of cancer are survivable. We use the most powerful tools of medicine to combat the invading malignancy. When one approach fails, we turn to another. We do not hesitate to suggest treatments that leave the patient suffering. Any weapon is part of the medical armamentarium.

We know how to treat schizophrenia, too, but good treatment is often unavailable. Unfortunately, just as with cancer, lack of effective treatment early on leads to a diminishing chance of recovery. With schizophrenia, the single most important factor determining the success or failure of treatment is the duration of untreated psychosis.

But people suffering from this illness don't usually realize they're ill and deny it if it's pointed out. This strange lack of self-awareness applies to medical illnesses as well as mental illness. People with untreated schizophrenia die on average 20 years early due to refusal of medical care. This denial of reality can be so thorough that, in one case, a woman failed to notice that she was pregnant and, when she went into labor, had no idea of what was happening to her. After her baby was born, she vehemently denied that she'd given birth. Unfortunately, this lack of awareness is the rule with severe mental illness, and hospital treatment is often required at the outset of treatment. Even a brief hospitalization can be transformative, as it was with Amari after one week at John George Hospital, allowing for successful outpatient treatment.

Ironically, those who champion the disability model end up creating true disability, when once there was opportunity for recovery. The disability model, as articulated by Disability Rights California, among others, holds that the most important fact for psychotic persons stricken with schizophrenia is their status as "disabled." According to this view, people disabled by severe mental illness must be defended against even brief hospitalization for treatment of their illnesses, because hospitals are "institutions." Even one day of hospitalization is called "institutionalization" if it's for psychiatric treatment. That the cost of denying hospital treatment may be incarceration, certainly a form of institutionalization, is ignored. The fact that delay of treatment reduces the chance of recovery and that lack of proper treatment ensures permanent disability is not a worry for these civil rights lawyers.

These attorneys rely on the Supreme Court's 1999 landmark decision in *Olmstead v. L.C.* (U.S. Supreme Court, 1999), which held that the unjustified segregation of people with disabilities is a form of unlawful discrimination under the Americans with Disabilities Act (ADA).

However, a closer reading of that decision indicates that *Olmstead* refers to "unjustified" segregation and does not forbid the treatment of severely ill patients in psychiatric hospitals. Justice Ruth Bader Ginsburg delivered the majority opinion of the Supreme Court, concluding that, under Title II of the ADA,

> States are required to place persons with mental disabilities in community settings rather than in institutions *when the State's treatment professionals have determined that community placement is appropriate. . . . Some individuals, like L. C. and E. W. in prior years, may need institutional care from time to time to stabilize acute psychiatric symptoms. . . .* The ADA is not reasonably read to impel States to phase out institutions, *placing patients in need of close care at risk. . . .* This Court emphasizes that nothing in the ADA or its implementing regulations condones termination of institutional settings *for persons unable to handle or benefit from community setting.* (U.S. Supreme Court, 1999; italics mine)

It seems clear that the Supreme Court recognized the need in some cases for hospital treatment ("institutional care") for people disabled by mental illness when denying such care would put them at risk and when they were unable to "handle or benefit from community setting." The court also concluded that the treatment professionals could be trusted to make such judgments.

The onset of psychosis is shattering for the young person and their family. Early intervention programs are their best hope, and the sooner treatment is begun, the better the chances of a stable recovery.

The signs and symptoms of oncoming psychotic illness have been extensively studied by schizophrenia researchers (Miller, McGlashan, and Rosen, 2003). The following are examples of symptoms that might herald a psychotic illness such as schizophrenia. It's important to keep in mind that no one sign or symptom by itself can predict the onset of this illness. Rather, it is the number and severity of such signs.

The good news is that during this prodromal phase of the illness, the young person still has insight and can recognize that something is wrong. With this insight, he or she is much more likely to accept help than later on, when the illness progresses and such insight often disappears. With these caveats, some signs that might predict later psychotic illness include:

- Unusual thoughts or delusional ideas
- Feeling persecuted or suspicious of previously trusted friends or family
- An exaggerated feeling of self-importance
- Perceptual abnormalities—for example, seeing flashes or fleeting visons of animals not seen by others or hearing sounds that others don't hear (e.g., phone ringing, sounds on the roof)
- Disorganized communication—having trouble making oneself understood, and having difficulty following conversations with others
- Loss of pleasure in social activities; feeling unhappy being around others, difficulty being at school; general withdrawal from family and friends

- Odd behavior and appearance, bizarre thinking
- Decreased personal hygiene
- Decreased functioning at school or work
- Trouble with focus and attention
- Difficulty sleeping
- General inability to feel pleasure
- Difficulty coping with normal stress

The subjects for this research were in their teens; the average age was 15. Normal adolescence is apt to be full of turmoil and change, and young people go through phases of unhappiness and difficulty adjusting more often than not. The point of these studies is not to label people as doomed to mental illness, but to help families who witness their adolescent children in unusual distress. If in fact a child is heading for a psychotic illness, it is important to begin intervention as soon as possible, for the family as much as for the child. Such specialized early treatment can enable healing and prevent the worsening illness that we see with delayed treatment. Early intervention in psychosis programs relies on a team of professionals who collaborate on care (RAISE, National Institute of Mental Health).

Good treatment takes much more than medication. It requires a coordinated program of individual therapy, family involvement, medication management, and a prompt return to work or school. One-on-one therapy with a skilled therapist helps the young person to cope with this shocking development. Psychotherapy helps to sort out the real from the unreal. Families need emotional support and education and to be included in the treatment program. Families are the single most important resource these young people have as they work to put their lives back together. Medication must be worked out carefully, over time, between patient and doctor, first to find the right drug then the lowest possible dose of that drug. Meanwhile, the doctor follows the patient with the rest of the team. Finally, the young person needs to regain his or her identity as a functional member of society, which means a return to school or work as soon as possible.

Schizophrenia has a lot in common with juvenile diabetes. Juvenile diabetes isn't preventable, but it is treatable. Treatment requires insulin; we have no other medication for type 1 diabetes. But with proper medical care, young people learn to manage their illness and care for themselves and to come to terms with the fact of this illness. Likewise, proper treatment early on helps young people with schizophrenia learn how to manage their illness. Over time, they become better able to sort out reality from delusion. They become more adept at sensing relapse and heading it off. They learn how to use the medications offered and to recognize their beneficial effects, especially in quieting the vicious hallucinations they suffer. And they learn how to advocate for themselves with their doctors. I saw all of that with Chris, whose mother brought him to my office in Walnut Creek.

The early intervention programs are the closest we come to prevention in the treatment of schizophrenia. They can't prevent the illness, but they provide intensive treatment during the early stages. Based on research done at the National Institute of Mental Health and developed by those researchers, this approach makes a significant difference in the course of this psychotic illness (Dixon, Srihari, and Kane, 2018; Lieberman, Dixon, and Goldman, 2013). Insel terms this approach "coordinated specialty care" (Insel, 2022; 186–89).

Unfortunately, these programs are not plentiful in the United States. Dixon and colleagues note that the United States is far behind Europe, both in research and in the development of necessary programs to provide this treatment (Dixon, Srihari, and Kane, 2018). They note, too, that American laws require the young person to deteriorate to the point of disability in order to qualify for Medicaid, which is often required to finance early intervention programs. Meanwhile, the illness worsens, and the prognosis becomes less hopeful with each passing month.

Insurance coverage is difficult to find. Despite the convincing studies documenting the effectiveness of early intervention, American insurance providers claim they don't have enough evidence that such programs work. While this rule may be profitable for the insurance companies, it is penny-wise and pound-foolish for taxpayers. Each person disabled by schizophrenia requires a lifetime of support: in disability payments, police time when they end up homeless, and prison expenses when they end up behind bars.

And this is only dollars and cents. The tragic cost is the loss of a meaningful life.

LACK OF HOSPITAL BEDS

Although the movement to shut down our mental hospitals is often seen as a triumph of civil liberty over oppression, it has exacted a cost. The people who bear this cost are those cursed with severe mental illness and their families. Many would say that the public pays the price, as well, as we struggle with the challenge of widespread homelessness.

The large state hospitals began to discharge patients after Thorazine became available. Although highly imperfect, this drug was the first effective antipsychotic medication, and many of the first people who left those hospitals were able to do so because of Thorazine.

But the main reason for the rapid closure of nearly all our mental hospitals was the IMD exclusion, which forbids the use of Medicaid to pay for treatment in a hospital that devotes more than half its beds to psychiatric care. After 1965, when the IMD exclusion took effect, patients were discharged regardless of whether they were ready and without a realistic plan for their care. We saw a flood of homeless people camped out on our streets, and for many, the prisons became their new home.

Today we continue to lose psychiatric hospital beds, and again money is the driving force behind this ongoing loss. A recent example is HCA Healthcare, a for-profit company with 186 hospitals and more than 2,000 freestanding sites of care, including surgery units, emergency rooms, labs, and urgent care centers across the country. HCA has a net worth of $74.14 billion, and it ranks 66 on the Fortune 500. But this summer, claiming it could not staff the unit, it closed its very small psychiatric service at Mission Oaks in San Jose as well as the pediatric intensive care unit.

Neither psychiatric care nor pediatric intensive care are lucrative, and a for-profit corporation must answer to its shareholders before any other consideration. These closures undoubtedly made business sense. But corporate ownership of medical care is increasing, and we should expect to see more shutdowns driven by the need for profits above all else.

SAMHSA

In 1992, the Substance Abuse and Mental Health Services Administration (SAMHSA) was carved out of Health and Human Services, with billions of dollars to fund its activities (Jaffe, 2017; 97–110). But the treatment of severe mental illness has not been part of its mission. For 20 years, there were no psychiatrists or other doctors on the board of directors or on staff, meaning no one with expertise in the medical treatment of schizophrenia or bipolar disorder. After 20 years, one psychiatrist was hired but left two years later, citing hostility to medical psychiatry.

SAMHSA was established to address mental illness. Although it has a Division of Prevention and Traumatic Stress, there is no mention of severe mental illness. Schizophrenia, which affects one out of every hundred human beings, is not mentioned. Neither is bipolar disorder. Neither one is preventable; they are brain disorders, and neither is caused by stress, even traumatic stress.

SAMHSA has programs to address "stigma," but studies show that stigma is not what gets in the way of treatment. Lack of availability is a far more important cause (Jaffe, 2017; 88). The closest it comes to early intervention in psychosis programs is a referral service, but it does nothing to support such programs and has no comment on their lifesaving function or their scarcity.

MENTAL HEALTH PROFESSIONALS OFTEN UNFAMILIAR WITH SEVERE MENTAL ILLNESS

Severe mental illness, a category including schizophrenia and severe bipolar disorder (bipolar I), is poorly understood by the general public. Amazingly, this goes for many mental health professionals as well. Severe mental illness is often not covered in graduate programs preparing students for a career in the field of mental health. Graduates preparing for their state licensing exams must complete thousands of hours of practical experience in the field. But the requirement for experience with severe mental illness is vague. State licensing exams often have no questions about severe mental illness.

This is a tragic situation. We need to revolutionize our approach to people with severe mental illness. We need to recruit more psychiatrists, but we also need to attract many more psychologists, psychiatric social workers, and other therapists to join in this effort. Treatment of the severely mentally ill requires a collaborative approach in which clinicians from the different disciplines work as a team. For that to work, each one needs to arrive on the job with an understanding of severe mental illness and a commitment to its treatment.

Finally, we need to make sure that everyone in this effort is well paid. Every professional should be paid as a professional. This work is important but challenging, and every clinician treating this most deserving population should be well compensated for their work.

COLLABORATION AND SENSE OF A COMMON MISSION

Collaboration among all the clinicians involved in caring for each client is essential to the care of our disabled patients. An example of good collaboration is the case of Morgan, who stopped all his medication and came to believe that his roommate was practicing witchcraft on him. What made all the difference for Morgan was that his case manager, Chloe, was a diligent communicator. She made a point of updating me on our mutual clients at the end of each day. When I brought up my concerns about Morgan, she reminded me of his past history of assault. Chloe had cultivated a good relationship with Morgan's house manager, who called her as soon as Morgan began acting strange. Deputy Ramos was a familiar and trustworthy presence who could work with all of us to help Morgan. In the end, it was easy for us to rectify the problem with his medications and help him get back his old volunteer job, which was important to his well-being.

Collaboration with case managers is not always so good in my experience. What I think of as the clinic at Dry Valley is not technically a clinic; it is a "service center." We had no case conferences of the sort where treatment is discussed. Our staff meetings were friendly but entirely devoted to social work issues, with a nursing report by Mei from

Good Hope Medical, addressed specifically to the case managers. The receptionists, who knew our clients well, were never invited. For me and the other psychiatrist, the staff meeting was entirely optional.

Chloe saw Morgan's problems as intimately related to his mental illness, an illness that was treatable. But often our case managers saw their role as limited to finding housing and benefits for their disabled clients. Even Lauren, our very able and hardworking clinic director, shrugged it off when Erik stopped his medication, despite his history of severe psychotic illness and life-threatening violence.

Most of our caseworkers are devoted and work diligently—many on their own time—to care for their clients. But the fact that our clients' disabilities stem from treatable mental illnesses is something our caseworkers were not always comfortable discussing. It's too bad, because we psychiatrists, who only see our patients for brief periods of time in our offices, can greatly benefit from the caseworkers' feedback about how our treatments are working.

Deborah, the confident and experienced caseworker who made a practice of listening to her clients as "part of their medicine," protested when I acceded to her client's wishes and changed the client's medication from injectables to pills. She worried that her client wouldn't take those pills, and she was right. The patient became acutely psychotic. Luckily, Deborah didn't hesitate to tell me about this development. I changed the prescription back to injectables, and the patient became lucid again.

This kind of direct collaboration is invaluable and should be the rule, not the exception. Housing our clients is part of their health care, but freeing them from psychotic states that get them ejected from their housing is part of their housing care. We need to understand that we have a common mission.

The case managers do have a common mission and work together to house their clients and to care for their health needs. They collaborate in formal case conferences and informally with other case managers. This sense of a common mission is invaluable to the work itself and to maintaining good morale, which is crucial in this challenging work. The caseworkers help their clients to get lifesaving financial support, housing, and health care. They care for their clients in the same way that parents care for their children's health needs. They ferry them to doctors' appointments as called for and to see their psychiatrists as required.

Communication in a medical setting has been systematically studied (Mundt et al., 2015). In 2015, researchers from the medical schools at Wisconsin and Northwestern looked at social connectedness on 31 teams at six primary care clinics. They asked each staff member (nurses, doctors, clerical workers, lab techs, and administrators) which of the other staff members they spoke with on a daily basis. In some offices, there was a high degree of interconnection, with most staff members speaking daily with many others on the same team. On other teams, which the researchers labeled "highly centralized," staff members tended to speak to a few central authority figures every day but not to each other. The researchers scored daily face-to-face communication separately from daily email contacts.

The results were striking. Patients cared for by the more socially connected teams did significantly better than those cared for by the highly centralized teams, as indicated by their significantly lower blood pressure and cholesterol levels. In addition, the more socially connected teams saved money, as their patients spent fewer days in the hospital and had fewer urgent care and emergency room visits.

It seems that friendly chats facilitate good patient care. Communication by email made no difference one way or the other. Contact had to be face-to-face to create this beneficial effect. Finally, the teams with a high degree of interconnection and collaboration also enjoyed the sense of a common mission.

I remember one receptionist at Dry Valley, Destiny, who was always aloof with me, unlike the others, who were easy to talk to. All of us ran into each other often in the mail room, so there was plenty of opportunity to make friendly connections. I kept looking for a way in with Destiny, though, until one day she said something about her vacation. It gave me the opening I was looking for, and she seemed to suddenly get that I wanted to have a more cordial relationship with her. After that, we enjoyed an easy rapport, and when she noticed that I needed something, she created it for me.

What I needed was personalized appointment slips to give my patients, with my name, number, and spaces for the time and date. She made me a large supply, printed on blue paper, enough to get through months of patients. It was so kind and so observant. And it started with a social chat about vacations.

INFORMATION AND MISINFORMATION: EMRS

Today electronic medical records (EMRs) have replaced our old SOAP records (subjective, objective, assessment, and plan—the standard format for writing medical notes). Computerized records can be a blessing if they're used for patient care. But in many settings, the EMR is used first and last as a billing tool. What we write in the medical record goes straight to the insurer—in our case, to Medi-Cal and Medicare. (The stringent HIPAA law makes a blanket exception for medical information sent to insurance companies.) Each patient visit is now a "unit of service," documented on a rigid computer form, the same form for each visit, no matter whether it's the first time we see a patient or one of many, with little new information to record. We spend as much time on our computers, documenting service for insurance billing, as we do with our patients.

Often we don't record information that doesn't fit in the insurance-oriented computer form, such as considerations of different diagnoses. We lack important information, such as long periods of high functioning, which tends to preclude a diagnosis of schizophrenia, or any information suggesting that the underlying problem is chemical dependency. Or, as with Marvin, my note lacked the most meaningful piece of information—the fact that he was too sick to come to the clinic and actively hallucinating to the point that he couldn't bear to speak with me.

After I began work at the Dry Valley clinic in Oakland, and later at the full-service partnership (FSP), I noticed that almost all my patients carried a diagnosis of schizophrenia in the EMR. Often that diagnostic code seemed wrong, but it was generally understood that checking that code on the form guarantees the highest insurance payment from Medi-Cal or Medicaid.

When I told this story to a physician friend who worked in emergency medicine, he was nonchalant. "Upcoding," he said. "We do that all the time."

Often I *could* make a more accurate diagnosis, but no one could tell me how to change the diagnosis in the EMR. My coworkers said, "That's the InSyst diagnosis," as if that explained why it was written in stone. So we wrote our EMR notes knowing that we were helplessly perpetuating a falsehood for the sake of insurance reimbursement.

We were instructed not to write substance abuse as the primary diagnosis, because Medi-Cal would refuse payment. But some of my patients suffered from severe addictions, which could very well have been causing all of their symptoms. Mr. Van Dyke, for instance, the man who lived under the freeway, was most likely abusing methamphetamine, and I doubt he'd ever suffered from schizophrenia. But driven by the InSyst diagnosis of schizophrenia, he was being prescribed a hefty dose of antipsychotics.

Likewise, Brandon, who wanted to be homeless, was abusing alcohol and heroin and clearly suffered from a mood disorder. But he was diagnosed as schizophrenic and treated with antipsychotics, which never helped him. I thought he needed rehab before anything else.

I could see that many of my patients were most likely not schizophrenic. Some suffered from mood disorders. Some were taking street drugs that made them look psychotic, but they probably didn't suffer from schizophrenia, meaning they most likely should not have been taking the powerful antipsychotic medications they were prescribed.

If I had the chance to get to know them well enough, I could discontinue those inappropriate drugs, as I had with Gracie. But at Dry Valley and still more so at the FSP, I often had to wait for weeks or even months before seeing a patient at a follow-up visit. So if I mistakenly stopped an antipsychotic drug that was actually working to stave off a psychotic episode, I would never know about it until way too late. This is one of the major benefits of treatment in an acute care hospital, where patients are safe even off their medications and where we see our patients every day and can monitor the effects of medication changes.

We were required to attend conferences instructing us on documentation and coding, but meetings to discuss patient care were rare and entirely optional. Although no one would have said it out loud, it seemed that our mission was first to keep the agency alive by diligently completing our service documentation.

One day we received a memo from our quality assurance (QA) officer at Dry Valley (QA seemed like a euphemism for making sure our documentation would guarantee payment). She sent us a long list (20 single-spaced pages) of common abbreviations—some medical, some part of our everyday language, such as "24/7." We were not to use any of these abbreviations without spelling them out first. If we failed to spell out these terms, the claim would be denied.

Obviously, this would add even more time to our documentation chores. And it seemed outrageous that the people passing judgment on our treatment decisions were so ill-informed about common medical terms (and ordinary English). I wrote to all the QA officers in the organization, asking why we couldn't just give that list of abbreviations to the reviewers, so they could look up a term themselves if they didn't understand it. The higher-ups never answered, and our QA officer simply wrote that it was "best practice." I wanted to write back and say, "No, it's worst practice," but I knew she was saying what she was told to say.

The reason for this bizarre directive became clear when I learned that some claims are reviewed by robots instead of human beings, based not on patient care but on profit. As BobKocher and Anuraag Chigurupati write in the *Journal of the American Medical Association*, "Health care organizations are applying new technologies like remote process automation and artificial intelligence. . . . A common use [of AI] is to manage prior authorization requests [sent from the doctor to the insurance company requesting that the recommended treatment be paid for by insurance]. A common administrative use for artificial intelligence is to assist with coding [for diagnosis and description of service] because the software can learn from payment and denial experiences [which] codes maximize revenue" (Kocher and Chigurupati, 2021). Upcoding is baked into the system.

And it seems that on each end, computerized algorithms are deployed: by the provider organizations to maximize payment and by the insurance companies to minimize payment. No wonder we have to spell out common abbreviations. The robots stumble over everyday language. So one wonders: how can they possibly understand the complexities of medical care? Yet it seems that robots are deciding which treatment, if any, is warranted.

Recently I spoke with Duane Brookhart, a PhD psychologist turned business analyst, with a specialty in medical business (Brookhart, 2023). When I asked him about upcoding, he said, "Upcoding is a euphemism for fraud."

But he added another story about systemic fraud, this time on the part of the medical insurance companies. In medical business analytics, he explained, a screener looks for fraud based on the organization's profit margin. "Several years ago," he wrote, "I analyzed a behavioral health group [four psychiatrists, two pediatric nurse practitioners, and several counselors] and was surprised by the fact that the profit margin was so low (the lowest I had ever seen in any medical specialty). I couldn't believe it, so I ran the numbers again and got the same result. Some insurers were essentially paying the provider nothing, and the providers were needing to subsist on the patient copays." He went on to explain that insurers can boost their business by listing mental health care as one of their covered benefits, and because they never plan to pay for it, that promise costs them nothing.

This has certainly been my experience and the common experience of my colleagues, which is why we are reluctant to see patients on their insurance. Word on the street is that we won't take insurance because insurance pays too little, but I doubt people realize that insurance often pays nothing. We are working for copay only, which is generally less than minimum wage.

The use of EMRs for insurance claims generates other misunderstandings. For example, it's often said that we psychiatrists are more apt to diagnose schizophrenia among Black patients than other patients, because of a racist distortion in how we see our Black patients. Perhaps this is so. Certainly schizophrenia is more commonly diagnosed in Black patients than in the rest of the population.

But the numbers can't tell the whole story. Our patients in these public clinics like Dry Valley and the FSP are overwhelmingly Black. Like all of our patients, they come to our public clinics because they can't afford anything else. People with means can more readily access private care. But in our clinics, all our patients are automatically diagnosed with schizophrenia regardless of their real illness. They come to us psychiatrists with their diagnostic label in place, conferred on them at intake by their case managers and locked into the computer system.

Unfortunately, this often repeated conviction is used as evidence that schizophrenia is not a real illness to be addressed with compassion and care in the Black community as elsewhere, but rather a racist "label" assigned by psychiatrists. I worry that it's used to undermine treatment.

There is no transparency and therefore no accountability in the EMR billing system. Clinicians and patients alike are at the mercy of a system that is completely opaque, so we have no way to challenge its methods or results. With the damage that this system causes to patient care, this is a system in desperate need of reform.

Many of us find it demoralizing when we can't give our patients adequate care. We suffer from moral hazard and go numb or else we leave. There is high turnover among the staff, which is bad for the patients and for the staff left behind. It leads to a feeling that what we're doing is pointless and that no one cares.

When a colleague of mine, one of our most able and dedicated social workers, finally left our clinic, she told me, "It's the hours of documentation added to my day, every day. And I feel like I'm telling a lie." No doubt she was referring to the meaningless boilerplate that ends up on the EMR form, with a fictitious recital of plan for improved behavior and the client's progress toward that goal. "And nobody reads them, anyway," she added.

She's right—most of us don't read the EMR notes. I would page through the EMR notes to glean what I could of a patient's history and response to treatment. But most of the notes were clearly copied and pasted from the same standard model to fill the boxes on the InSyst form without revealing anything about that particular patient. It's understood that these documents are for the benefit of the Medi-Cal and Medicare reviewers.

The problem is not that records today are digital rather than on paper. If the goal is patient care rather than billing, useful computer records can be created and organized so that clinicians can find what they need with a few clicks on the keyboard.

The problem is not the EMR per se. It's that we're also locked into a fee-for-service system, which sets up an escalating struggle between clinicians and insurers over payment. When the EMR record serves as a billing document, we clinicians are forced to spend as much time documenting service as we do with our patients.

At first I thought this destructive situation was limited to our sector—the care of poor people with mental illness. Then in 2020, as the COVID-19 pandemic ramped up, Siddhartha Mukherjee published a story in the *New Yorker* about the EMR (Mukherjee, 2020). He had begun to receive alarming reports of blood clots in COVID patients. But when he turned to our multibillion-dollar EMR system to look for similar reports and find patterns in the data, he was stymied. He and others resorted to social media to communicate their findings. They also shared their exasperation with the EMR system. Mukherjee describes one such exchange.

> A cardiologist at Massachusetts General Hospital, in Boston, echoed this frustration on Twitter: "Why are nearly all notes in Epic [a major supplier of EMR systems] . . . basically *useless* to understand what's happening to patient during hospital course?"
>
> Another doctor's reply: "Because notes are used to bill, determine level of service, and document it rather than their intended purpose, which was to convey our observations, assessment, and plan. Our important work has been co-opted by billing."

A cardiologist at Mass General, the nation's most prestigious medical center, was experiencing the same frustration with the EMR as we were.

I realized the insanity of this setup wasn't limited to mental health care, or to poverty clinics, or to Alameda County.

Finally, Mukherjee comments on the time wasted by our EMR system. "We've been saddled with systems that cut into patient care (clinicians typically spend an hour feeding documentation into a computer for every hour they spend with patients)," he writes.

PSYCHIATRISTS UNABLE TO PROVIDE PROPER CARE

Psychiatrists in public clinics often see very little of their most severely ill patients. Our chief function is often limited to renewing prescriptions for patients we barely know and signing off on disability claims. For our very sick patients, a brief office visit every three months is considered adequate. This is drastically insufficient. Combined with our lack of usable medical records, it leads to dangerously insufficient patient care.

Although some would argue that psychiatric diagnosis has no place in mental health care and that diagnosis is simply an oppressive "label," in reality it's important to good patient care. We need to know if the patient has a severe mental illness requiring medication in addition to psychotherapy. And if medication is needed, which medication? The answer starts with an accurate diagnosis. We need to know if chemical dependency is complicating the picture or if it's actually the main issue. We need to know if psychotherapy alone is appropriate, in which case diagnosis fades into the background, as good psychotherapy is not focused on diagnosis.

Accurate diagnosis is important when the problem is severe mental illness. Not all psychosis is a result of severe mental illness. We have to rule out "organic" causes, meaning medical illnesses that cause psychosis. These range from drug toxicity to thyroid disorder to metastatic cancer with metastases to the brain and a host of other possibilities. Certain symptoms, such as visual or olfactory hallucination, are "organic" until proven otherwise.

My experience is that all of us would love to discover some unusual cause of what looks like a common illness—in med school we'd hear "good pickup" from our teachers if we managed this feat. But more often we'd hear, "When you hear the sound of hoofbeats, don't think of a zebra." Nevertheless, we longed to be that star diagnostician who found the zebra.

In reality, the most common causes of psychosis in our work are schizophrenia, bipolar disorder with psychotic symptoms, and drug toxicity. At first, though, these can all look alike. If they're available, good medical records can help to sort this out.

It used to be that the medical "note" (what clinicians wrote in the hospital record, whether on paper or electronically) was a document dedicated to patient care. In that note, we wrote what the patient told us (subjective), what we observed (objective), our assessment (assessment), and our treatment plan (plan). The mnemonic is SOAP. The note was as long or as short as it needed to be—a page or more for a new patient and as little as several lines for an ongoing progress note. After the patient was discharged from the hospital, we'd write a discharge summary: a page or more documenting the course of treatment, final diagnosis, and recommendations for further treatment, as necessary. When we saw a new patient in the hospital or in the clinic, we would review the previous notes in the medical record. Past medical records could tell us which approaches succeeded, which failed, which diagnoses were considered or rejected. Then we left our own notes in the record for those who would come after us.

The medical record was a means of organizing our thinking and communicating with other clinicians caring for the same patient. All this is lost, of course, when the medical note is used as a billing document.

Combining medical notes with billing turns the computer template into a procrustean bed: we mangle and truncate our reports to fit into arbitrary boxes on the screen. No wonder the Mass General cardiologist complained that hospital progress notes were useless.

In the world of good care, psychiatrists see new patients for follow-up shortly after their initial visits, a week or less if the illness is severe. We need to see patients often enough to get to know them and to let them get to know us. This means genuine conversation. We need to keep an open mind to look for signs of health and strength that we might have missed and also for signs of difficulty that we might have missed.

Meanwhile, the patient makes their own determination: *Does Dr. Feller seem like the right person? Does she know what she's doing? Can she be trusted? Do I like her?*

If we're using medication as part of the treatment, we need to hear whether it was useful. Did it help with sleep or anxiety? Did it stop the voices? Is the patient actually taking the new drug? If the medicine stays in the bottle, we need to know that and why it's staying in the bottle. Did it have noxious side effects? Is it scary? Does it feel like mind control? If my patient doesn't trust me, I'll never hear about any of this.

We also need to know what other mind-altering drugs the patient is using. Street drugs, medical marijuana, and alcohol can cause problems with mood and cognition. If the patient is taking significant amounts of methamphetamine, for example, he or she may be suffering from amphetamine psychosis or severe depression brought on by withdrawal. Alcohol in excess can cause depression and even be implicated in suicide attempts. Cannabis in any form, including medical marijuana, can cause or prolong depression and in rare cases precipitate psychotic episodes.

But I won't hear about any drug use unless the patient senses that I'm actually interested in his experience. That takes listening, and listening takes time. A treatment limited to prescriptions of antipsychotics or other medication is drastically inadequate.

If the patient is acutely psychotic and too delusional to use outpatient treatment, hospital treatment can provide safety and a chance to stabilize. In the safety of the hospital, we can take our patients off all their medications, allow street drugs to clear from their systems, and see who they are at baseline. This was the case with Betsy, my patient on Ward 2N. We were able to hold off on giving her antipsychotic drugs because in the hospital we could keep her safe. We collaborated on our assessment of her situation, and when I presented her in our case conference, others recognized the signs of amphetamine psychosis.

The fact that she and I had gotten to know each other helped, too. She felt comfortable enough, once she was drug free, to tell me about the Ritalin. I felt free to discharge her from the hospital as soon as she was back to normal after that last conversation.

Transparency and Accountability

There were many times, when I worked at the FSP and at Dry Valley before, that I remembered Sophie's story about the administrator who told her, "Sophie, no one's going to sue you." Communication and transparency are crucial for accountability, but our system of mental health care lacks transparency and is short on communication regarding medical treatment. An absence of accountability is the result.

In many areas of medicine, the threat of lawsuit helps to safeguard patients against negligent care. Many hospitals have morbidity and mortality review boards to examine cases in which patients suffered unexpectedly bad outcomes so that clinicians can learn from their experiences. But as our administrator told Sophie, no one in our system gets sued, no matter how egregious the negligence. We saw this with Lucille, who lost her life at San Geronimo Hospital. Often our patients have no one to advocate for them.

In settings where clinicians collaborate on patient care, the natural oversight that occurs when colleagues work together acts as a safeguard. We see each other's work. It's not just that we took an oath to do no harm; we want to be able to hold up our heads and keep our jobs. But in my recent experience of public mental health care, collaboration on treatment is the exception, and sloppy care is often the result.

Lack of collaboration can be fatal, as with my patient Patrick. When I tried to look back at how we'd failed in his care, I found that his record had been expunged from the system. There was no way for us to look together at how we had failed him and to learn from our mistakes. With Lucille, who died due to casual neglect at San Geronimo Hospital, we all knew it was gross negligence. We were the only ones who would advocate for her, yet we were apparently barred from doing so, allegedly to protect her confidentiality.

HIPAA

On February 15, 2022, the Berkeley City Council held a special meeting to address homelessness and severe mental illness in the city. A number of speakers complained about the privacy laws that interfere with communication among agencies caring for the homeless and mentally ill.

They were referring to HIPAA, the Health Insurance Portability and Accountability Act of 1996, a federal law meant to safeguard the confidentiality of electronic medical records (Jaffe, 2017; 196–98).

The law requires that clinicians do what we've always done: obtain our patient's permission before sharing information with another clinician caring for that patient. It allows for exceptions for medical necessity.

For my private practice, I created a special form for this purpose, a two-way release. When I ask for permission and present my patients with the form for their signature, I have never been refused. I've never been refused by a clinic patient, either. People seem glad that their providers collaborate on their care. Sometimes they request that we do so.

HIPAA was never meant to be a tool of secrecy or an excuse to avoid collaboration. Nevertheless, it is frequently cited as a reason for not sharing vital information among individuals or agencies caring for the same person.

Worse still, HIPAA is used as an excuse to refuse family members the opportunity to speak to us about their loved ones. Family members are our patients' most valuable allies and have important information to give us. Nothing in HIPAA or elsewhere bars us from listening to family members or others; we don't ever need permission to listen. Unfortunately, this is often unclear to clinicians and other staff, who refuse to listen when family members have information to impart.

I've seen claims of confidentiality used to bar family members from contact with their lost loved ones. Family members are excluded from writ hearings, those legal proceedings held on-site, which decide whether their loved ones remain in the hospital. Families have no opportunity to alert clinicians and judges to facts that would bear on the legal decision. Often the result is that the patient is discharged from the hospital while still desperately in need of care. Parents, unaware of the hearing, aren't informed about their child's imminent discharge. They have no chance to go to the hospital and meet with their son or daughter and bring him or her home. Often patients are simply discharged to the street, with no arrangement for follow-up care. Although the medical necessity exemption clearly applies for these acutely ill patients, administrators claim that HIPAA requires this cruel practice.

An atmosphere of guardedness pervades our mental health system, to the great detriment of everyone, especially our patients.

FRAGMENTED SYSTEM: NONPROFITS AND THE MILLIONAIRES TAX

Our system of mental health care in California is highly fragmented. Part of what makes it so is a function of Proposition 63, which passed in 2004 and created the "millionaires tax," meant to fund mental health care in California. Prop 63 dictates that all the money raised by this tax must be funneled through nonprofit agencies. Each nonprofit is separate from all the others, with no mandate to communicate or cooperate on patient care.

In many ways the nonprofits function like small businesses. They must compete with one another for the same funding—Prop 63 revenue and county, state, and federal funds. Often several agencies provide the same services to the same population. This was the case when I worked at the FSP and our agency suddenly lost the representative payee function to another nonprofit agency, which meant our case managers could no longer issue checks to their clients. Although our case managers were supposed to be providing social services for our clients, a competing agency also was providing social services to the same clients and had been given that valuable tool.

In 2015, when the Little Hoover Commission, an independent state oversight agency, set out to assess how well Prop 63 funds were being used, they ran into a wall of obfuscation. Transparency was rare, making accountability nearly impossible. They couldn't tell how well Prop 63 was working or whether it was mostly a failure. They cited a few instances in which things were going well but conceded that the rest was a mystery (Little Hoover Commission, 2015).

Another example of fragmentation is the relationship between Dry Valley and Good Hope Medical. At Dry Valley, we shared common space with the Good Hope Medical Clinic next door to us. Although their patients were already our patients, referred to Good Hope by us for medical care, and although any Good Hope staff member could log into our EMR and read our patients' psychiatric records, we were not allowed to log into the Good Hope system to see our own patients' medical histories—to check on things we needed to know, like what medications they took and what medical problems they suffered. Sophie told me the reason for this was that Good Hope felt we couldn't be trusted to respect patient confidentiality.

As a favor, the Good Hope clinic director, Mei, would print out the record of the patient's latest Good Hope Clinic visit before we saw a patient, unless she forgot or unless there wasn't enough lead time. It was always understood that she was doing us a favor.

When writing a prescription, you should know what other drugs a patient is taking and any medical problems they might have. Otherwise, for all you know, you're giving your patient a drug their body can't handle due to other medical problems, such as kidney or liver insufficiency. Or you unwittingly prescribe something that causes a toxic drug interaction. We could ask them, of course, but even the most clear-thinking people are often unable to name all the medications they take and to remember correctly all their medical history. For our patients, these questions are impossible to answer with any degree of reliability. We need their medical records.

In a unified system, this would never have been tolerated. If both of our agencies had been part of the same system, we could have complained about the dangerous nature of this setup to someone higher up in the system. But there was no higher authority that oversaw both our clinics. Good Hope staff reported to Good Hope administrators, and we reported to Bay Area Community Service, two separate nonprofits contracted with Alameda County.

Occasionally I sent my patients to the Good Hope doctors for medical consults, a common practice between clinicians in any healthcare setting. The consultant can send a written response or, in a setting where all the clinicians see each other often, the consultant might buttonhole the referring clinician to discuss the patient briefly. When I first arrived at Dry Valley, I'd conferred with Dr. Jones at Good Hope about a mutual patient, a typical "curbside consult." Always, when you send a patient for consultation, you identify yourself as the referring doctor.

But I realized that I didn't have the email addresses of the doctors at Good Hope. I would know which doctor followed my patient, but

I couldn't copy him or her on the consult I sent to Good Hope. It felt unprofessional and not very collegial. I thought it was something that had fallen through the cracks, as I had many other clinicians' email addresses throughout the county system.

I asked Mei, the Good Hope clinic director, if I could get their email addresses so that I could copy the Good Hope doctors on my consult requests. She refused. "Our doctors don't have time to talk to you," she explained.

I ran into Sally, our departing clinic director who overlapped with Lauren, and asked her if there was some way around this. "We'll take care of it," she said.

When I handed in my resignation, I gave my boss two months to find a replacement for me. It was just as I was about to leave that I got a brief message with the Good Hope doctors' email addresses. One of the doctors wrote back to me promptly. "It's about time," he said. I expect he'd been wondering why the consults from our clinicians remained anonymous.

In the meantime, I talked to Lauren, who told me her own story. After a laborious effort to arrange a medical appointment for one of our clients, she emailed the client's primary care doctor (not a Good Hope doctor) to let her know. Instead of thanking her, the doctor wrote back and blasted Lauren for writing. "You shouldn't have my email address," she said.

It was inexplicable. In a well-functioning system, we would all have each other's contact information.

On a routine basis, this fragmentation, the isolation of one nonprofit from all the others, leads to waste and duplication of effort. It stymies our efforts to take good care of our patients. Each of us works as if at the bottom of a deep hole, unable to look out and see our neighbors, let alone collaborate on patient care.

THE QUESTION OF HOSPITAL TREATMENT

In 2021, Disability Rights California (DRC) brought a lawsuit against Alameda County Behavioral Health (ACBH), alleging that it was mistreating its disabled citizens who suffered with severe mental illness. It "relies too heavily on institutional care" for this population, DRC wrote. Federal law requires disabled people to be cared for in the community, it claimed, in the "least restrictive setting." Hospitals are institutions, which for the purpose of disability law, are not "in the community." DRC was crusading to end hospital care for our patients, although deinstitutionalization had nearly accomplished that job already. Of course, the institutions we do rely on are jails and prisons, but DRC ignores this reality.

The lawsuit was heavily covered in the local press and even in the national press. The *San Francisco Chronicle* quoted Aaron Fischer, who was cocounsel on the lawsuit. "I call it a 'coin toss,'" he said, "whether you end up in the jail or the psychiatric facility" (*San Francisco Chronicle*, 2021). When I called him to ask if he really meant that jails and psychiatric facilities were the same, he said he did.

I find it ironic that these professional disability lawyers fight to maintain the status quo, a system that leaves their clients disabled for life and often truly institutionalized behind bars. If they really wanted to help their disabled, severely mentally ill clients, they would fight for early intervention in psychosis programs and enough hospital beds to care for their clients. Instead, their actions keep their clients homeless or locked away behind bars, becoming increasingly more disabled as time goes on.

Nevertheless, these rather uninformed lawyers have the loudest voices in the debate over how best to treat severe mental illness, although a few others speak out in opposition. Some of these are people with lived experience of severe mental illness and its treatment. Jason Park is one of them who compared his very good hospital experience in Pittsburgh, Pennsylvania, with that in California (Park, 2023). Another is Patricia Wentzel, a peer advocate and case manager for NAMI Sacramento, who also serves on the Sacramento County Mental Health Board. Recently she wrote in *CalMatters* about her personal experience (Wentzel, 2023).

"My own involuntary hospitalizations have been like wearing steel-toe boots without the right socks. They slid around a little, but my toes were protected," she writes.

As she regained her sanity in the hospital, she saw the same "miracle" in her fellow patients: "The catatonic returned to life, the utterly fearful, restored to trust, the fearless saved from ruin and certain death—I witnessed these transformations in locked wards. I have seen sanity restored where there was only despair, delusion, rictus grins or silent stares." Some were healed through standard treatment, others by the place itself.

In 2022 I attended a meeting with DRC and US Department of Justice attorneys (who joined the lawsuit) to discuss their claims. The DOJ attorney who spoke reiterated their position. Avoiding "institutional" care was the most important issue, she said. People disabled by severe mental illness (SMI) could get everything they need without hospitalization, she said, if only ACBH provided sufficient outpatient treatment. She ignored the fact that unawareness of being ill and the resulting refusal of treatment are part of severe mental illness. "Gentle, consistent persuasion," she said, was all that was needed to get these disabled folks into treatment. And housing, she added. "Housing first" was key. She seemed unaware that people who suffer from SMI often walk away from board and care or family homes because of ongoing psychosis (auditory hallucinations and delusional states). She ignored the fact that lack of hospital care leaves many people with SMI locked up in prison and truly institutionalized.

Present at the meeting were a number of family advocates, mothers whose adult children had lived with untreated SMI for years. They begged for more hospital beds. They know through bitter experience that their children have no idea that they're ill and this lack of self-awareness is part of the illness.

One by one they described their children's desperate straits—those who had survived so far. Their sons and daughters lived in prison or on the streets, homeless for years and often self-medicating with meth, fentanyl, and other street drugs. These parents lived in fear, dreading the phone call that would inform them of their missing child's death.

Sometimes they lived in fear for their own lives, too. Many slept behind locked doors. Katy Polony, an in-home outreach team (IHOT) member, helps her client families draw up a safety plan for use if necessary:

- Keep your phone with you at all times.
- Lock your bedroom door.

- Put away the knives or other potential weapons.
- Make sure you can exit a room. Don't get trapped.
- Alert the neighbors of the situation and recruit them as allies. Encourage them to call 911.
- Be proactive. Let the police and crisis teams know the situation.

At that meeting, the mothers repeated what is common knowledge among these families but was unknown to the general public, much less to the civil rights attorneys: when the situation in the home becomes dangerous and the police are called, they generally refuse to help facilitate hospitalization (possibly because there are no beds in the hospitals). Instead, they tell the desperate mother that she needs to take out a restraining order against her child and kick them out of the house. It's known as "streeting," as the young person inevitably winds up on the streets.

If the son or daughter tries to return to the family home, the parent is to call the police to complain that the child is violating the restraining order. At that point, the police will arrest the young person and take him or her to jail. Although beds in the hospital are nearly impossible to come by, there are always beds in the jail. Needless to say, following these directives may damage the parent-child relationship beyond repair.

These parents had tried everything, of course, for years, including gentle, persistent persuasion. Housing was never the issue. Their children were not living on the streets for lack of housing. It was their untreated mental illness that put them in such danger.

After each parent spoke, the DOJ attorney said, "I hear you" or "I feel your pain," and repeated her arguments. She recommended the FSP approach, adding that FSPs were known as "hospitals without walls." Perhaps some people believe this. But I thought, listening to her, of the FSP where I had worked. Where the case managers searched in vain for their clients, and where I'd met only a few of my patients. Where the others were never found.

One of the many cruelties heaped on these mothers is blame for their children's illnesses, a common myth with no basis in fact. At the first and subsequent meetings with her IHOT families, Polony tells them: "You are not to blame, there is no shame, and you are not alone." Often her words bring tears of relief.

Epilogue

Suggestions for Change

1. Abolish the IMD exclusion and restore hospital care for acute psychosis and other mental health crises and residential treatment for people of all ages struggling with chemical dependency. The Lanterman-Petris-Short Act in California and similar laws in other states provide strict limits on involuntary commitment; there is little chance of patients being forgotten and left indefinitely in hospitals. But too often our patients with severe mental illness end up locked away behind bars, forgotten by all but their families.

2. Early intervention in psychosis programs, modeled on the RAISE (Recovery After an Initial Schizophrenia Episode) protocol, should be standard treatment for anyone with a first episode of psychosis. Proper care early on saves lives and money. Insurance should be required to fully cover this treatment.

3. Students in all psychology, clinical social work, and counseling programs should receive instruction about major mental illness and hands-on experience with this population. Include major mental illness on state licensing exams for professionals specializing in mental health care, including masters programs in social work and marriage and family therapy and doctoral programs in psychology.

4. Require SAMHSA to devote the majority of its funds to the treatment of severe mental illness and to reserve a majority of the seats

on its board for psychiatrists and other clinicians with deep expertise in the treatment of severe mental illness.

5. End the practice of delegating mental health care to nonprofit organizations, and instead provide this care in one unified system, such as the statewide system common outside California. This would foster communication, transparency, and accountability; cut down on turf wars; and save money.

6. Reassess and clarify the HIPAA law so it can't be used to exclude families from contact with their loved ones, to deny properly requested medical records, or to avoid communication among professionals caring for the same patient.

7. Institute morbidity and mortality review boards in the mental health system so that clinicians can learn from their mistakes and work together to improve care.

8. Permanent supportive housing is desperately needed. Board and care homes must be funded well enough to serve as high-quality permanent supportive housing.

9. Require large private nonprofit healthcare systems to provide acute and subacute inpatient psychiatric care for adults, at levels commensurate with community needs, as a condition of maintaining their nonprofit status. Require the same of for-profit healthcare systems as a condition of maintaining their licenses to operate.

10. Use electronic medical records for patient care only, and leave billing to others, such as clinic administrators. Restore the SOAP (subjective, objective, assessment, and plan) format to medical notes, with accurate diagnostic codes and detailed intake and discharge summaries. Never deny properly authorized requests for medical records.

11. Structure treatment teams to encourage collaboration among team members across disciplines, with leadership to foster such collaboration.

12. Create a directory of services, up-to-date and available to every clinician in each public health jurisdiction (county in California, state elsewhere), listing all mental health, chemical dependency, and housing services in that jurisdiction. Include which services are provided, which insurance is accepted, and a contact person reliably available for inquiries by referring clinicians.

REFERENCES

Alexander, B. (2017). *Glass house: The 1% economy and the shattering of the all-American town*. St. Martin's Press.

Autur, D., & Hanson, G. (2013). The China syndrome: Local labor market effects of import competition in the United States. *American Economic Review, 103*(6), 2121–68.

Avalos, G. (2015, February 14). Turnaround in Downtown Oakland. *Mercury News*.

Bailey, Z., Feldman, J., & Bassett, M. (2021). How structural racism works—racist policies as a root cause of U.S. racial health inequities. *New England Journal of Medicine, 384*, 768–73. https://doi.org/10.1056/NEJMms2025396

Bion, W. (1962). *Learning from experience*. Basic Books.

Bion, W. (1967). Notes on memory and desire. The Psychoanalytic Forum, *2*(3).

Boedecker, E., & Dauber, J. (Eds). (1973). *Washington university manual of medical therapeutics*. Wolters Kluwer.

Boyer, L. B. (1956). On maternal overstimulation and ego defects. *Psychoanalytic study of the child, 11*, 236–56.

Brookhart, D. (2023). Medical business analytics. www.medicalbusinessanalytics.com.

Cahalan, S. (2012). *Brain on fire: My month of madness*. Penguin Books.

Cahalan, S. (2019). *The great pretender: The undercover mission that changed our understanding of madness*. Grand Central Publishing.

Case, A., & Deaton, A. (2020). *Deaths of despair and the future of capitalism*. Princeton University Press.

Clinton, B. (2000). Expanding trade, protecting values: Why I'll fight to make China's trade status permanent." *New Democrat, 12*(1), 9–11.

Conan Doyle, A. (1892). The adventure of the speckled band. *Strand Magazine*.

Curtin, S., & Hedegaard, H. (2019). Suicide rates for females and males by race and ethnicity: United States, 1999 and 2017. Division of Vital Statistics and Division of Analysis and Epidemiology, Center for Disease Control and Prevention.

Dixon, L., Goldman, H., Srihari, V., and Kane, J. (2018). Transforming the treatment of schizophrenia in the United States: The RAISE initiative. *Annual Review of Clinical Psychology, 14*, 237–58. https://doi.org/10.1146/annurev-clinpsy-050817-084934

Forman Jr., J. (2017). *Locking up our own: Crime and punishment in Black America.* Farrar, Straus and Giroux.

Franceschi, C., & Campisi, J. (2014). Chronic inflammation and its potential contribution to age-associated diseases. *The Journals of Gerontology: Biological Sciences and Medical Sciences, 69*(S1), S4–9. https://doi.org/1093/glu057

Freud, S. (1894). The neuro-psychoses of defense. In *The Standard Edition of the Complete Psychological Works of Sigmund Freud* 3 (pp. 45–61). Hogarth Press Limited, 1966.

Freud, S. (1895). On the grounds for detaching a particular syndrome from neurasthenia under the description "anxiety neurosis." In *The Standard Edition of the Complete Psychological Works of Sigmund Freud* 3 (pp. 87–115). Hogarth Press Limited, 1966.

Freud, S. (1896a). Heredity and the aetiology of the neuroses. In *The Standard Edition of the Complete Psychological Works of Sigmund Freud* 3 (pp. 141–58). Hogarth Press Limited, 1966.

Freud, S. (1896b). Further remarks on the neuro-psychoses of defense. In *The Standard Edition of the Complete Psychological Works of Sigmund Freud* 3 (pp. 159–85). Hogarth Press Limited, 1966.

Freud, S. (1912). Recommendations to physicians practicing psycho-analysis. In *The Standard Edition of the Complete Psychological Works of Sigmund Freud* 12 (pp. 115). Hogarth Press Limited, 1966.

Geronimus, A. T., & Thompson, J. P. (2004). To denigrate, ignore or disrupt: Racial inequality in health and the impact of policy-induced breakdown of African-American communities. *Du Bois Review, 1*(2), 247–79.

Geronimus, A. T., Hicken, M., Keene, D., & Bound, J. (2006). "Weathering" and age patterns of allostatic load scores among blacks and whites in the United States. *American Journal of Public Health, 96*(5), 826–33. https://doi.org/10.2105/ajph.2004.060

Gladwell, M. (2008). *Outliers: The story of success*. Little, Brown and Company.

Goodwin, D. W. (1977). *Adoption studies on alcoholism*. University Press of Kansas.

Greenberg, J. (1964). *I never promised you a rose garden*. Holt, Rinehart & Winston.

Grotstein, J. S. (1977). The psychoanalytic concept of schizophrenia: I. The dilemma and II. Reconciliation." *International Journal of Psychoanalysis, 58*, 427.

Grotstein, J. S. (1980). A proposed revision of the psychoanalytic concept of primitive mental states: I. Introduction to a newer psychoanalytic metapsychology." Contemporary Psychoanalysis, 16(4), 479–546.

Grotstein, J. S. (1989). A revised psychoanalytic conception of schizophrenia: An interdisciplinary update." *Psychanalytic Psychology, 6*, 253–75.

Grotstein, J. S. (1990). The "black hole" as the basic psychotic experience: Some newer psychoanalytic and neuroscience perspectives on psychosis. *Journal of the American Academy of Psychoanalysis, 18*(1), 29–46.

Gundersen, S. (2022). Psychoanalysis and neuropsychological explanations. *Psychoanalytic Review, 109*, 415–37.

Hays, P., & Tilley, J. R. (1973). The differences between LSD psychosis and schizophrenia. *Canadian Journal of Psychiatry* (August 1).

Insel, T. (2022). *Healing: Our path from mental illness to mental health*. Penguin Press.

Jaffe, D. J. (2017). *Insane consequences: How the mental health industry fails the mentally ill*. Prometheus Books.

Janowsky, D. S. (1976). Marijuana effects on simulated flying ability. *American Journal of Psychiatry, 133*(4): 384–88.

Kendler, K. S., & Diehl, S. R. (1993). The genetics of schizophrenia: A current, genetic-epidemiologic perspective. Schizophrenia Bulletin, 19(2), 261–85.

Kesey, K. (1962). *One flew over the cuckoo's nest.* Viking Press.

Kimball, W., & Scott, R. (2014). China trade, outsourcing and jobs. *Economic Policy Institute.* https://epi.org/publication/china-trade-outsourcing-and-jobs/

Kindy, K., Fisher, M., Tate, J., & Jenkins, J. (2015, December 26). A year of reckoning: Police fatally shoot nearly 1,000. *Washington Post.*

Knoebel, R., Starck, J., & Miller, P. (2021). Treatment disparities among the black population and their influence on the equitable management of chronic pain. *Health Equity, 5*(1), 596–605. https://doi.org/10.1089/heq.2020.0062

Kocher, B., & Chigurupati, A. (2021). economic incentives for administrative simplification. *JAMA, 326*(17): 1681–82. https://doi.org/10.1001/jama.2021.18292

Ksir, C. (2016). *Cannabis and psychosis: A critical overview of the relationship.* National Institutes of Health.

Lidz, C. W., Meisel, A., Zerubavel, E., Carter, M., Sestak, R., & Roth, L. H. (1984). *Informed consent: A study of decision-making in psychiatry.* Guilford Press.

Lieberman, J. A., Dixon, L. B., & Goldman, H. H. (2013). Early detection and intervention in schizophrenia: A new therapeutic model." *JAMA, 310*(7), 689–90.

Lieberman, Jeffrey. (2023). *Malady of the mind.* Simon & Schuster.

Little Hoover Commission. (2015). Promises still to keep: A decade of the mental health services act. Report #225. https://lhc.ca.gov/report/promises-still-keep-decade-mental-health-services-act

Marshall, M. (2011). Early intervention for psychosis. *Schizophrenia Bulletin, 37*(6), 1111–14.

Massey, D. S. (2007). *Categorically unequal: The american stratification system.* Russell Sage Foundation.

Messman, T. (2016, August 8). *Street spirit.* https://issuu.com/streetspirit/docs/2016-08-august-street-spirit

Miller, T., McGlashan, T., & Rosen, J. (2003). Prodromal assessment with the structured interview for prodromal syndromes and the scale of prodromal symptoms: Predictive validity, interrater reliability, and training to reliability. Schizophrenia Bulletin, 29(4), 703–15. https://doi.org/10.1093/oxfordjournals.schbul.a007040

Mishel, L., and Bivens, J. (2017). The zombie robot argument lurches on." *Economic Policy Institute*, May 24. https://files.epi.org/pdf/126750.pdf.

Morrisette-Thomas, V. (2014). Inflamm-aging does not simply reflect increases in pro-inflammatory markers." *Mechanisms of Ageing and Development, 139*, 49–57. https://doi/org/10.1016/j.mad.2014.06.005.

Mukherjee, S. (2020, May 4). What the coronavirus crisis reveals about American medicine. *New Yorker.*

Mundt, M., Gilchrist, V., Fleming, M., Zakletskaia, L., Tuan, W.-J., and Beasley, J. (2015). Effects of primary care team social networks on quality of care and costs for patients with cardiovascular disease. *Annals of Family Medicine, 13*(2), 139–48.

Rosenfeld, H. (1987. *Impasse and interpretation*. Routledge.

Rosenhan, D. L. (1973). On being sane in insane places. *Science, 179*, 250–58.

Sandel, M. (2018, May 9). Populism, Trump and the future of democracy. *OpenDemocracy*. https://opendemocracy.net/en/population-trump-and-future-of-democracy/

Sandler, J. 1960. The background of safety. *The International Journal of Psychoanalysis, 41*, 352–56.

San Francisco Chronicle. (2021, April 26). Justice dept. blasts mental health care. B1.

Scott, R. (2000). The high cost of the China–WTO deal: Administration's own analysis suggests spiraling deficits, job losses. Economic Policy Institute. Issue Brief #137.

Scull, A. 2023. Rosenhan revisited: Successful scientific fraud. *History of Psychiatry, 34*(2). https://doi.org/10.1177/0957154X221150878

Searles, H. 1976. Psychoanalytic therapy with schizophrenic patients in a private-practice context. *Contemporary Psychoanalysis, 12*, 387–406.

Simons, R. L., Lei, M.-K., Beach, S. R. H., Barr, A. B., Simons, L. G., Gibbons, F. X., & Philibert, R. A. (2018). Discrimination, segregation, and chronic inflammation: Testing the weathering explanation for the poor health of black Americans." *Developmental Psychology, 54*(10), 1993–2006. https://doi.org/10.1037/dev0000511

Social Security Administration. (n.d.). Frequently asked questions (FAQs) for representative payees. www.ssa.gov/payee/faqrep.htm?tl=11

Szasz, T. (1961). *The myth of mental illness*. Harper and Row.

Thurman, R. (Ed.) (1977). *Alcohol and aldehyde metabolizing systems*. Volume 3: *Intermediary metabolism and neurochemistry*. Elsevier Academic Press.

Torrey, E. F. (2012). *The insanity offense: How America's failure to treat the seriously mentally ill endangers its citizens*. W. W. Norton & Company.

U.S. Bureau of Labor Statistics. (n.d.) Concepts and Definitions. www.bls.gov/cps/definitions.htm

U.S. Supreme Court. (1999). *Olmstead v. L.C.*, 527 U.S. 581. https://caselaw.findlaw.com/court/us-supreme-court/527/581.html

Vaillant, G. E. (1977). *Adaptation to life*. Little, Brown and Company.

Vaillant, G. E. (1995). *The natural history of alcoholism*. Harvard University Press.

Vedam, S., Stoll, K., Khemet Taiwo, T., Rubashkin, N, Cheyney, M., Strauss, N., McLemore, M., Cadena, M., Nethery, E., Rushton, E., Schummers, L., Declercq, E., & GVtM-US Steering Council. (2019). The giving voice to mothers study: inequity and mistreatment during pregnancy and childbirth in the United States. *Reproductive Health, 16*(77).

Waldinger, R. J. (1973). The study of adult development. http://hr1973.org/docs/Harvard35thReunion_Waldinger.pdf

Washington Post. (n.d.). 994 people shot dead by police in 2015. www.washingtonpost.com/graphics/national/police-shootings/

Wentzel, P. (2023, September 18). Coercion for the mentally ill in California can also be a form of compassion. *CalMatters*.

Winnicott, D. (1965). Ego integration in child development. In *The Maturational Processes and the Facilitating Environment* (pp. 56–63). International Universities Press.

Zaheer, J. (2020). Predictors of suicide at time of diagnosis in schizophrenia spectrum disorder: A 20-year population study in Ontario, Canada." *Schizophrenia Research, 222*, 382–88.

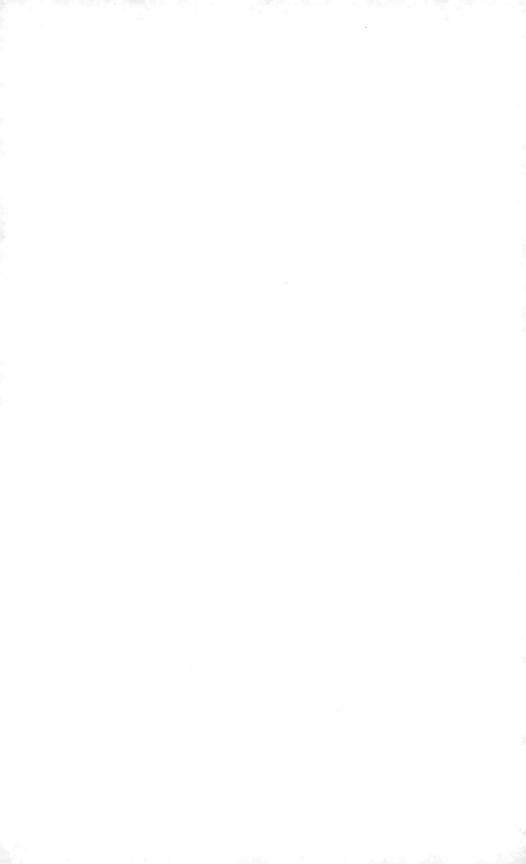

INDEX

About the Author

Alice Feller, MD is a writer and a clinical psychiatrist. After graduating from medical school at the University of Pittsburgh, she completed her psychiatry residency at UC San Francisco and a physician fellowship in substance abuse treatment at the San Francisco VA Medical Center. She has worked in private practice, hospital emergency rooms, psychiatric wards, chemical dependency programs, and public mental health clinics. Her writing, focused on mental health, addiction, and homelessness, has appeared in the opinion pages of the *New York Times* and the *San Francisco Chronicle* as well as the *East Bay Express*, the *Laney Tower*, *CalMatters*, *fort da*, and *Interconnecting Circles*. She lives with her husband and daughter in Berkeley, California. She served two terms on the City of Berkeley Homeless Commission and is an analyst member of the San Francisco Center for Psychoanalysis.